Planning for the Found

Ideas for themes and activities

Penny Tassoni

Heinemann Educational Publishers,
Halley Court, Jordan Hill, Oxford OX2 8EJ
A division of Harcourt Education Ltd

Heinemann is a registered trademark of Harcourt Education Limited

OXFORD MELBOURNE AUCKLAND JOHANNESBURG BLANTYRE GABORONE IBADAN
PORTSMOUTH NH (USA) CHICAGO

First published 2002
2006 2005 2004 2003 2002
10 9 8 7 6 5 4 3 2 1

A catalogue record for this book is available from the British Library on request.

ISBN 0 435 40167 X

Typeset by 𝍤 Tek-Art, Croydon, Surrey

Printed and bound in East Lothian by Scotprint

Websites
Please note that the examples of websites suggested in this book were up to date at the time of writing.
It is essential for tutors to preview each site before using it to ensure that the URL is still accurate and
the content is appropriate. We suggest that tutors bookmark useful sites and consider enabling students
to access them through the school or college intranet.

Tel: 01865 888058
www.heinemann.co.uk

For two very special friends: Nora and Frances

Contents

How to use this book

The Foundation Stage curriculum has been widely applauded by many early years experts, but many practitioners have found the size and layout of the curriculum guidance folder to be daunting. This book is designed to guide practitioners and students through the Foundation Stage curriculum guidance and provide them with ideas of themes and activities that will bring the curriculum to life.

The book is divided into two sections:

Part 1 Understanding the Foundation Stage

This section begins by considering the aims and purpose of the Foundation Stage curriculum and explores the layout of the folder. It then guides practitioners and students through each of the areas of learning, focusing in on some of the key points that underpin the curriculum guidance and suggesting ways of meeting children's needs. To assist in the planning of each of the areas of learning, checklists of activities, layouts and routines are provided.

Part 2 Themes and activities for the Foundation Stage

To help practitioners and students plan for the Foundation Stage, this section contains twenty carefully chosen themes. Each theme is based on the idea that children learn most effectively from direct experiences and that themes are best used as starting points that can be adapted to meet children's needs and interests. The themes are presented in traditional 'spider web' format as many practitioners will use this style when planning. Each theme is accompanied by six activity plans, one for each of the areas of learning. The activity plans detail the key learning intentions, resources required, as well as the role of the adult. They also show how the activity links to other areas of learning in the Foundation Stage curriculum. Ideas to vary and extend children's learning are also presented so that practitioners and students can capitalise on children's enthusiasm and interests.

Acknowledgements

I would like to begin by thanking Mary James and Anna Fabrizio at Heinemann for their continued support and patience. I would also like to thank Jennifer Enderby, Gill Heseltine, Gail Holderness and Louise Burnham for giving of their time and expertise and for allowing me to tap into their wealth of experience.

I would also like to thank the many practitioners, college lecturers and students who, through their positive comments and feedback, help to shape my work.

Finally, another 'Thank you' to the Tassoni team who continue to support me in countless ways.

Penny Tassoni
August 2002

The author and publisher would like to thank the following individuals and organisations for permission to reproduce photographs and copyright material: Gareth Boden pages 19, 22, 25, 26, 30, 36; Haddon Davies pages 14, 33; QCA/DfES page 3; Gerald Sunderland pages 7, 9; Taxi/Ron Thomas page 16.

Every effort has been made to contact copyright holders of material published in this book. We would be glad to hear from unacknowledged sources at the first opportunity.

Part 1 Understanding the Foundation Stage

Background to the Foundation Stage

The Foundation Stage curriculum was introduced in England in September 2000. It is a curriculum for children aged three to five years who are in settings that receive the nursery education grant.

The Foundation Stage curriculum is regarded by many involved in early years education as a landmark, indicating a return to play-based learning for children. Concerns had been growing that young children were being expected to start their formal education before they were physically and emotionally ready. Evidence from European and other countries that delay formal education until children are six or seven years old was increasingly drawn upon to show that successful learning outcomes in reading, writing and number skills did not depend on an early formal start, but rather upon the readiness and maturity of the child. The previous early years curriculum, entitled 'Desirable Learning Outcomes', and the related inspection process, was criticised for pressurising pre-schools and nurseries into starting formal education and reducing the emphasis on learning through play. A change of approach was clearly needed. Therefore, the creation of a 'stage' to reflect that early childhood play experiences are important in themselves has been well received, as have been the opportunities for wider training and support for early years practitioners.

Key features of the Foundation Stage
- Recognition that young children need to learn through practical experiences rather than being taught.
- Play is emphasised as the vehicle of learning for children.
- The importance of working from children's interests and needs is highlighted.
- It is the first curriculum in England to cross the divide between pre-school and schools.
- Personal, social and emotional development of children is recognised as providing the backdrop for other learning.
- The role of parents is promoted as that of being an equal partner.

Curriculum guidance for the Foundation Stage

The curriculum guidance for the Foundation Stage is published by QCA (Qualifications and Curriculum Authority). It is presented in the form of a ring binder or folder and is therefore often referred to as 'the folder'! It is available free of charge from QCA (see p. 41 for the contact details). It is important that each member of staff, helper or student has his or her own copy of the guidance as OfSTED, the inspection body, will expect adults in your setting to have a good working knowledge of its contents. The section on curriculum guidance in this book aims to help you find your way around the guidance, but you will need a copy of the guidance itself to refer to.

Structure of the folder

A good starting point is to familiarise yourself with the structure of the folder. The folder is divided into three main sections:

1 The Foundation Stage

This introductory section looks at the aims of the Foundation Stage.

2 Principles of early years education

This short section looks at the principles of the Foundation Stage and indicates how these principles should be put into practice in your setting. Note that among the principles is the idea that this curriculum is play-based and also child focused.

3 Areas of learning and Early Learning Goals

The rest of the folder looks at the curriculum. This is divided into six areas of learning. This part of the folder must be used when planning activities and experiences for children as otherwise you run the risk of missing out significant parts of the curriculum.

Looking at areas of learning

The areas of learning make up the majority of the folder.
   There are six areas of learning:

- Personal, social and emotional development
- Communication, language and literacy
- Mathematical development
- Knowledge and understanding of the world
- Physical development
- Creative development.

Tip It can be difficult when using the folder to find the area of learning that you are looking for. Consider buying or making a set of dividers!

Each area of learning contains an introduction, which gives practitioners examples of information about what they should aim to provide and teach children. Once past the introduction, you will find a series of double-page spreads. The pages are divided into four colours. Each colour represents a stage. There are no 'definite' ages attached to each stage. This is deliberate: you should consider what children are able to do, rather than simply their date of birth. If you are new to working with the Foundation Stage and children in it, you may find the table below helpful, though remember that children do not always fit into neat bands!

Yellow	– Children in this stage are likely to be the youngest children, that is, very young three year olds.
Blue	– Children in this stage are likely to be older three year olds/very young four year olds.
Green	– The stage at which many children will be starting their reception classes.
Grey	– By the time most children are in this stage, they are likely to have completed their reception year. The early learning goals are in this band as they are goals of the reception year.

Looking at a double-page spread

These are the steps that children need to pass on the way to the Early Learning Goal.

This section is designed to help you think about children's stages of development. You may see children in your group playing in the same kind of ways.

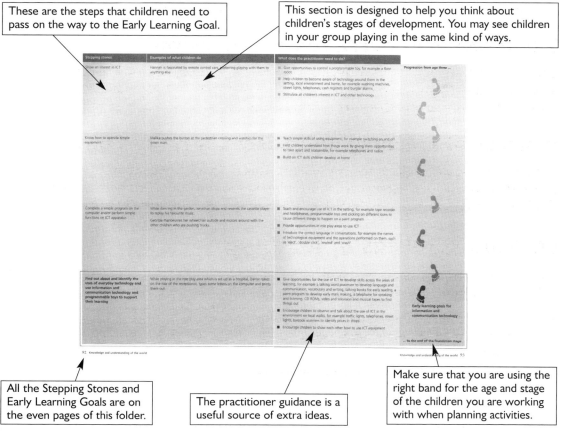

All the Stepping Stones and Early Learning Goals are on the even pages of this folder.

The practitioner guidance is a useful source of extra ideas.

Make sure that you are using the right band for the age and stage of the children you are working with when planning activities.

Left-hand page – This shows the Stepping Stones and Early Learning Goals together with accompanying examples of what children in each stage might do.

Right-hand page – This gives some examples of how practitioners might work with and support children.

Aspects of learning

Each area of learning is subdivided into aspects of learning. This is not immediately obvious in the folder, but is referred to in further guidance produced by QCA in 2001 entitled 'Planning for learning in the Foundation Stage'. The aspects of learning are very useful to refer to when planning. They ensure that you are covering each area of learning fully. The table below shows the aspects of learning along with the page reference in the curriculum guidance.

Area of learning	Aspects of learning	Curriculum guidance page
Personal, social and emotional development	Disposition and attitudes Self-confidence and self-esteem Making relationships Behaviour and self-control Self-care Sense of community	32 34 36 38 40 42
Communication, language and literacy	Language for communication Language for thinking Linking sounds with letters Reading Writing Handwriting	48, 50, 52, 54 56–8 60 62 64 66
Mathematical development	Numbers as labels and for counting Calculating Shape, space and measures	74 76 78–80
Knowledge and understanding of the world	Exploration and investigation Designing and making skills Information and communication technology Sense of time Sense of place Cultures and beliefs	86, 88 90 92 94 96 98
Physical development	Sense of space Movement Health and bodily awareness Using equipment Using tools and materials	104 106, 108 110 112 114
Creative development	Exploring media and materials Music Imagination Responding to experiences, and expressing and communicating ideas	120 122 124 126

How to interpret the areas of learning

Personal, social and emotional development

This is the first area of learning in the curriculum guidance for the Foundation Stage. It is considered to be an essential area of learning for all children, hence its prominent place in the guidance. As practitioners it is important that we do not gloss over this area, as children who leave us feeling confident, motivated, secure and aware of others are more likely to fulfil their potential and succeed not only in formal learning but in life.

There are six aspects of learning.

Aspects of learning	Curriculum guidance page
Disposition and attitudes	32
Self-confidence and self-esteem	34
Making relationships	36
Behaviour and self-control	38
Self-care	40
Sense of community	42

Disposition and attitudes

In many ways this aspect of learning could be paraphrased as an 'appetite for learning'. We need to make children feel that learning is fun, challenging, exciting, and therefore worth concentrating on and persisting in.

Key messages in the Stepping Stones and Early Learning Goals

◆ **Concentration and perseverance** – should come from the child rather than being forced onto them. Note for example, that the green Stepping Stone suggests that children may persist with an activity of *their* choosing. This means that insisting children should 'sit' or join in with an activity is likely to be inappropriate.

◆ **Independence and exploration** – children will need time when they can choose their own activities and materials. We should also encourage children to 'explore' their own ideas, rather than just follow others.

Delivering this aspect of learning

On paper this may seem an easy aspect of learning to deliver, but in reality it is quite a challenge. It means looking carefully at the routine of the setting, the environment, and the support we are providing to make sure that we are not in any way ' boring' children or preventing them from taking the initiative.

Good practice checklist

◆ Are children able to choose, get out and put away resources?
◆ What proportion of the children's time is being spent simply 'waiting' or 'listening', e.g. at snack time, home time, start of the day?
◆ Are children's particular interests followed and encouraged?
◆ Do planned activities allow children to explore and be creative?
◆ Does the routine of the day allow children time to 'play' at self-chosen activities?
◆ Do adults praise children who have been playing, and therefore concentrating, for long periods?

Self-confidence and self-esteem

This aspect of learning is about children's feelings and understanding of self. If children are feeling good about themselves, they will find it easier to respect and think about others. Children who have such self-awareness by the end of the reception year will find it easier to co-operate with others and to cope with their feelings.

Key messages in the Stepping Stones and Early Learning Goals

◆ **Separating from main carer** – this is of prime importance as it affects children's sense of security.
◆ **Encouraging children to talk about home and their community** – will help children to develop a strong self-image.
◆ **Helping children to articulate their needs and feelings** – when children can 'label' their feelings and needs, it becomes easier for them to exercise some control.

Delivering this aspect of learning

The starting point must be to consider the effectiveness of your settling-in policy, as children who are not feeling secure will find it hard to manage their own feelings. It is no longer considered satisfactory for children to 'cry' for a few minutes at the start of a session. They should have made a sufficient attachment to an adult to be able to separate. Consider working intensively with those children who, after an absence or holiday, find it hard to settle in.

Good practice checklist

◆ Are times created for children to be in pairs or alone with their key worker so that they can build up a strong relationship?
◆ Do adults in the setting listen carefully and encourage children to talk about what they do at home?
◆ Are activities that may stimulate talk about home and community provided, e.g. home corner, doll's house and displays?
◆ Are activities provided so that children can hear language about feelings being 'modelled', e.g. a storybook about being angry or a puppet feeling sad?

Making relationships

This aspect of learning is about helping children to socialise and to co-operate with each other.

Key messages in the Stepping Stones and Early Learning Goals

◆ **Trust and making attachments** – the first Stepping Stone is about children feeling secure and becoming interested in others.
◆ **Coping with changes in routines** – this is about children being flexible and secure enough to cope with changes.
◆ **Sharing and turn taking** – note that this is hard for younger children and so is an eventual Early Learning Goal.

Delivering this aspect of learning

The ability to socialise and co-operate with others is partly a developmental process, which relies on children's language and cognitive skills. Understanding where children are in terms of the Stepping Stones and having realistic and fair expectations of individual children is therefore essential.

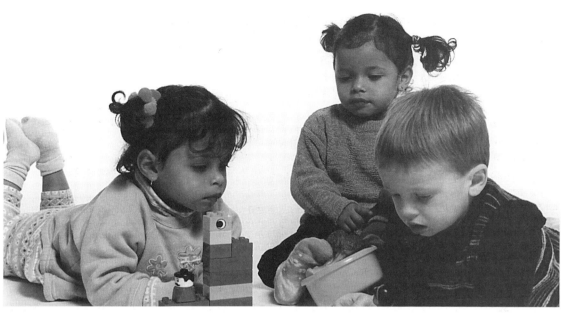

Is equipment put out that will encourage younger children to play alongside each other?

Good practice checklist

◆ Is equipment put out that will encourage younger children to play alongside each other?

◆ Are games and activities played in very small groups so that children can build up relationships?

◆ Do adults model the language that children will need to use so that they can join in with others, e.g. 'May I join in your game?'

◆ Do all the children know each other's names?

◆ Does the setting have a routine and are changes explained to children?

◆ Are children encouraged to problem-solve together?

◆ Does the setting encourage children to 'celebrate' together individual children's achievements, e.g. 'Let's all have a clap?'

◆ Do children understand the reasons behind certain 'rules' in the setting?

Behaviour and self-control

This aspect of learning focuses on children being able to think about others and adapt their behaviour accordingly.

Key messages in the Stepping Stones and Early Learning Goals

◆ **Right and wrong and consequences of actions** – note that it is only in the eventual learning goal that children should understand the consequences of their actions and words. The Stepping Stones towards this goal are about helping children to understand the needs of others and guiding them towards being aware of boundaries.

Delivering this aspect of learning

It is important not to interpret this aspect as 'getting children to do as they are told'. The focus is clearly on helping children to understand the needs of others and the need for certain boundaries. Self-control and understanding that others have needs is also tied to children's overall development. It is therefore particularly important that children with a developmental delay are worked with according to the Stepping Stone that best matches their stage of development.

Good practice checklist

◆ Are children encouraged to help with putting out activities and tidying up?
◆ Do children understand the context behind certain boundaries, e.g. 'If you throw sand, it may hurt another child', or 'If we all help to tidy up, we can play another game?'
◆ Do adults praise children when they show caring actions towards others?
◆ Are children listened to and encouraged to find their own solutions to situations, e.g. several children wanting to go on the slide at once?

Self-care

This aspect centres on children's growing ability to be independent. It links to children's confidence.

Key messages in the Stepping Stones and Early Learning Goals

◆ **Pride in achievements** – is in the first Stepping Stone. If children gain satisfaction from doing things themselves, they will be more motivated to concentrate and learn.
◆ **Initiative taking and choice** – are in each of the Stepping Stones and are the key features in this aspect.

Delivering this aspect of learning

The starting point for this aspect of learning is to look at your layout and routine. Children need easy access to resources and materials and to be encouraged to choose them. As adults working with children, we must also think about our role. For children to become independent and used to taking the initiative, we will sometimes need to 'hold' back and encourage rather than take over!

Good practice checklist

◆ Are basic resources, such as aprons, scissors, drawing materials, displayed for children's use?
◆ Are toys and equipment, such as funnels or measures, displayed for children's use?
◆ Do children have to ask permission before they take out materials or can they help themselves?
◆ Are children encouraged to put back the materials they have finished with?
◆ Is it possible for children to go to the toilet/wash their hands without asking first?
◆ How are children's efforts recognised when they attempt to do things for themselves, e.g. blow their own noses?
◆ Are children encouraged to help each other?

Sense of community

This aspect of learning is about children valuing themselves and others. It is closely tied to the 'Cultures and beliefs' aspect of learning in 'Knowledge and understanding of the world'.

Key messages in the Stepping Stones and Early Learning Goals

◆ **Sense of self** – the starting point for this aspect of learning. Children need to be confident about themselves in order to accept others.
◆ **Awareness of others' needs, beliefs and cultures** – comes in much later with children being expected just to know that others may not have the same beliefs, needs and cultures as they do.

Delivering this aspect of learning

This aspect of learning represents a change of direction in terms of how settings should be promoting equal opportunities. The emphasis now is on getting the child to recognise their own lifestyle before looking at those of others. It is no longer appropriate for young children to celebrate festivals from different faiths unless it has a particular meaning and relevance for a child or children in the setting.

The key to delivering this aspect of learning is therefore to find as many opportunities as possible for children to talk about things that are important in their lives, going to visit a favourite relative, their favourite food, their favourite clothes. It is also important that we show genuine interest and are positive about what children are telling us.

Good practice checklist

◆ Are there regular opportunities for children to talk to adults and their friends about different areas of their lives, e.g. birthday parties, weddings, food they eat?

◆ Are activities planned that help children realise that everyone has different likes, dislikes and feelings?

◆ Are activities planned that recognise individual children's lifestyles, e.g. the role-play area is made into an aeroplane because a child has recently been on holiday?

◆ Do resources, posters, equipment relate to children's home lifestyles?

◆ Are parents involved in the setting and is their expertise being used?

◆ Do adults show that they are positive, keen to learn and interested in others' experiences?

◆ Are activities/games planned where children have to find out information from each other, e.g. 'Find out if the child next to you has any brothers or sisters'; 'Find out if they have a teddy or toy that they take to bed'?

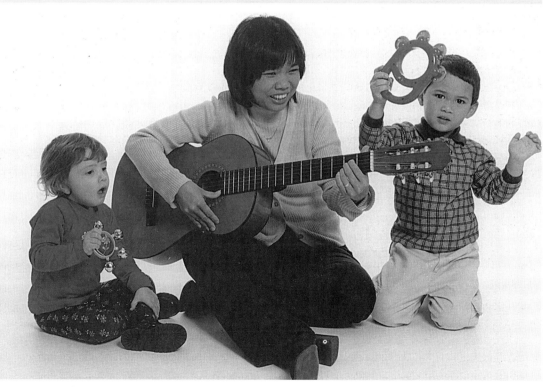

Are parents involved in the setting and is their expertise being used?

Specific activities for promoting personal, social and emotional development

Many of the Stepping Stones and Early Learning Goals for this area of learning can be promoted through the routine of the setting.

Putting out and tidying away resources and materials

Children can be put in small groups or 'teams' so that at the beginning or end of a session they work with an adult to tidy up specific areas of the setting. This structure means that children can be with their key worker and also get to work co-operatively with each other. By giving each 'team' a specific area, it helps children to gain a sense of achievement and avoids situations where some children tidy up but others learn how to avoid doing so!

Working alongside adults

It is important to find opportunities where very small groups of children can work with an adult, e.g. washing up and drying the snack-time beakers. These periods of time encourage children to talk individually with an adult whilst helping them to feel responsible. Looking for opportunities for children to join adults also helps children to learn specific skills, e.g. filing children's work, putting up a display, ordering from a catalogue. Parents may also be involved in this way, e.g. they may show children how to cook or bring in objects of interest. Traditionally this was a key way in which children learned skills and spent time with adults.

Puppets and cuddly toys

Puppets and cuddly toys provide a good way of modelling language to children so that they have the expressions and vocabulary they need to talk about their emotions and feelings. They can also be used to help children think about behaviour, e.g. teddy is sad because although he will not share his toys, he wants his friends to play with him.

Storybooks

There is a huge range of stories available that will help children to talk about their homes and feelings. As children are more likely to talk when they have the undivided attention of an adult, it is useful to look for opportunities for them to share stories in small groups or, when possible, individually with an adult.

Displays and interest tables

Displays of children's work help them to feel proud and valued. Where possible, children should be involved in actually putting up the display or choosing items for it. Displays that help value their homes and interests are essential, e.g. a display of children's favourite clothes, photographs of parties they have been to, or even favourite foods and recipes.

Valuing personal, social and emotional development

One of the key challenges when delivering this area of learning is to ensure that parents understand its importance. Many parents send their children to pre-school settings and into school expecting their children to learn. While they recognise the value of children's attempts at counting or writing, they may not automatically realise the importance of children helping to tidy up or being able to dress themselves and make choices and decisions.

◆ Videotape or photograph children as they are playing so that parents can see how they are learning to concentrate.

◆ Make sure that parents know when their children have played for extended periods of time.

◆ Praise children and make sure parents are aware when they have tried out a new activity.

◆ Work with parents to set some goals for each child involving self-care skills, e.g. being able to wipe their own nose, put on their coat, tidy away.

Activity – *Personal, social and emotional development*

Many parents are not aware of the link between personal, social and emotional development and their child's ability to learn.

Produce a leaflet for parents that explains the importance of this area of learning. Show how the routines and activities in your work setting provide opportunities to cover this area of learning of the Foundation Stage curriculum.

Communication, language and literacy

This area of learning encompasses speaking and listening as well as early skills in reading and writing.

There are six aspects of learning.

Aspects of learning	Curriculum guidance page
Language for communication	48, 50, 52, 54
Language for thinking	56–8
Linking sounds with letters	60
Reading	62
Writing	64
Handwriting	66

Language for communication

This first aspect looks at helping children to use language as a way of socialising and expressing their needs. It also includes encouraging children to listen.

Key messages in the Stepping Stones and Early Learning Goals

◆ **Interacting and speaking** (pp. 48, 52 – curriculum guidance) – the first Stepping Stones suggest that children will rely on simple gestures and words to make their meaning clear. The practitioner guidance looks at extending children's language by reflecting back what they want to say and giving opportunities to interact with other children with adult support.

◆ **Listening** (p. 50) – in the first Stepping Stone, children are only expected to listen when they are in one-to-one and small-group situations and when the conversation interests them. Being able to sustain listening is an Early Learning Goal, but note that it is active listening, with children able to respond with questions and comments. Listening is not about being quiet!

◆ **Vocabulary** (p. 52) – should be gained by hearing new words in context. The role of the practitioner in modelling language is emphasised. Note that the practitioner does not directly correct vocabulary, but models it back to the child correctly.

Delivering this aspect of learning

To deliver this aspect well, adults will need to spend time with children supporting and modelling language. With younger children this should be in one-to-one situations and in very small groups. Adults will need to model language for children, so providing a puppet or cuddly toy to act as a stooge will be helpful.

It is also important for all adults in the setting to understand that listening should be 'active' and that young children find it hard to listen and be quiet – they will need to respond to what is being said.

Good practice checklist

- ◆ Do children get regular opportunities to talk with adults on a one-to-one basis?
- ◆ Are puppets/cuddly toys used to model language?
- ◆ Do adults 'expand' young children's simple statements?
- ◆ Are adults allowing enough time for children to 'think' before responding?
- ◆ Are activities provided that encourage children to 'work' together in small groups?
- ◆ Are quiet times provided for individual children to be 'listened' to without interruption?
- ◆ Do adults act as good role models by listening to children?

Language for thinking

This aspect of learning recognises that language is linked to cognitive development. Children who have good language development find it easier to remember things and structure their thoughts.

Key messages in the Stepping Stones and Early Learning Goals

- ◆ **Talk** – this is of prime importance as children often need to 'talk' in order to organise their thoughts and to direct themselves.
- ◆ **Use language for imagination** – this appears in the last Stepping Stone and is one of the Early Learning Goals for this aspect. Children should be encouraged to predict, see patterns and think through scenarios.

Delivering this aspect of learning

Language for thinking requires children to explain, to describe their thoughts and use language to organise what they are doing. This requires quite a high level of language, so we must look for ways of modelling some of the language that they will need, e.g. games such as 'What do you think I have in my hand?' It is also important to respect children's need to talk aloud. Child development theory suggests that children are only able to internalise their thoughts fully when they are around six or seven years old. Discouraging them from talking aloud therefore tends to prevent them from thinking. The use of very small groups when carrying out activities is essential so that children can talk freely.

Good practice checklist

- ◆ Are regular games provided which encourage children to ask questions, e.g. 'Guess what is in the feely bag'; 'What do you think teddy bought in the shop today?'
- ◆ Do all adults in the setting understand the importance of children being able to talk aloud especially when something interests them?
- ◆ Are questions framed, which encourage children to think, e.g. 'Why do you think it is …?'
- ◆ Do adults build children's vocabulary by accurately naming items and feelings?
- ◆ Are activities planned, which will encourage children to work out patterns, predict what will happen next, e.g. 'What will happen if we mix the blue paint with the yellow?'

Linking sounds with letters

This aspect of learning covers the beginnings of early literacy. Being aware of sounds and letters will help children to both read and write later on. There is a clear emphasis on helping children to hear sounds of letters through the use of rhymes rather than 'letter of the week' type scenarios. This represents a change of approach from the previous early years curriculum.

Key messages in the Stepping Stones and Early Learning Goals

- **Distinguishing one sound from another** – this is in the first Stepping Stone and is important, as activities that help children to listen carefully will eventually help them to 'tune' into letter sounds.
- **Rhymes and rhyming activities** – the use of rhymes is in all of the Stepping Stones. This is to help children listen carefully to sounds in words. It is worth noting that this approach replaces the idea of learning about individual letter sounds.
- **Naming and sounding the letters of the alphabet** – this is an Early Learning Goal and therefore not expected of the youngest children or those still working on the Stepping Stones.

Delivering this aspect of learning

The starting point for this aspect of learning is to work on children's auditory discrimination by helping them to listen out for sounds and to notice the patterns and rhythm of words. Musical games, poems and rhyming stories can be used alongside nursery rhymes and songs to help children listen and tune into sounds in words.

> ### Good practice checklist
> - Do the adults in your setting know their traditional nursery rhymes?
> - Are parents aware of the nursery rhymes that are being learned in the setting?
> - Is there time set aside for children to sing and repeat nursery rhymes?
> - Is there a programme to ensure that children learn a range of nursery rhymes?
> - Have you a collection of simple poetry books for children to share with adults?
> - Are stories selected with rhythmical refrains for the children to join in, e.g. 'Trip, trap, trip, trap, who's walking on my bridge?'
> - Are games such as sound lotto regularly available for children to play?
> - Are there regular opportunities for children to play musical games, e.g. going on a bear hunt?
> - Do adults draw children's attention to the sounds in their names and in the environment, e.g. 'Smiling Susan – do you want to come and have a drink now?'

Reading

This aspect of learning concentrates on motivating children to read rather than an ability simply to decode. This is important because the desire to read and the love of books and other written materials is now recognised as playing a vital role in children's later successful reading.

Key messages in the Stepping Stones and Early Learning Goals

- **Listen to stories** – this is in the earliest Stepping Stone. Note that for young children it suggests that stories and poems should be shared on a one-to-one basis or in small groups. Therefore it is not appropriate to expect children on this Stepping Stone to listen to whole-group stories.

◆ **Have favourite books and learn how to handle books** – the enjoyment of books is key to this aspect of learning. The idea behind children having favourite books is that they will associate print with meaning whilst learning how to handle and use books. The green Stepping Stone suggests that children need a variety of books – this is important as many settings tend to stock more fiction than non-fiction books.

◆ **Read words** – the decoding of familiar and common words is expected as an Early Learning Goal. For most children this will be at the end of their reception year, many children, however, will be able to recognise their names and signs that have meaning for them before then.

Delivering this aspect of learning

Many settings find that parental pressure for children to formally learn to read is great. To avoid this, it is essential to work with parents so that they understand the importance of pre-reading skills. Make sure parents understand that the desire to read, as well as knowledge about how books 'work', is the basis for later successful reading. In some settings it may also be worth considering devising a checklist of pre-reading skills so that parents can see that their child is making progress.

It is also important that the routine of the setting is considered to ensure that children have time with adults when they can listen to a story by themselves or in very small groups. This close interaction allows children to handle and to turn the pages of books, ask questions and feel involved with the story. It also allows us to show children with our fingers how print in English runs from left to right.

Good practice checklist

◆ Can children freely access adults to share stories with them on a one-to-one basis or in pairs?

◆ Are stories chosen that have rhyming or repeated refrains?

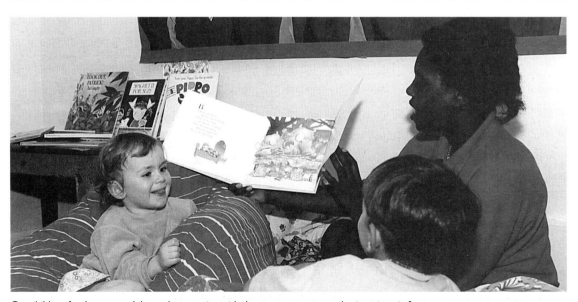

Can children freely access adults to share stories with them on a one-to-one basis or in pairs?

- Are children encouraged to take care of books, e.g. display them, place them carefully on a shelf?
- Are books attractive and suitable for the age of the children?
- Is there a variety of books including poetry, fiction, non-fiction?
- Are there plenty of signs in the setting and do adults refer to them, e.g. 'Can you remember what the sign says?'
- Are name cards used to help children recognise their names, e.g. posting them when they arrive in the setting?
- Can children take home 'favourite' books so that they can share them with their parents?
- Is a record kept of children's favourite books?
- Do children see adults reading in the setting, e.g. following a recipe, reading a letter?
- Do children sometimes get letters from adults in the setting?

Writing

This aspect of learning looks particularly at children's desire to communicate, at first using marks but eventually more recognisable letters. It needs to be read in context with reading and handwriting.

Key messages in the Stepping Stones and Early Learning Goals

- **Mark making** – this is the starting point for children's early writing, with children gradually becoming more purposeful and knowing what they are trying to write. Note that there is no mention of children copying down or tracing over words. The aim is that the writing should come from the child.
- **Begin to break the flow of speech into words** – the practitioner guidance suggests that we should be 'scribing' for children, e.g. writing in front of them what they would like to say. As children watch us do this, they will connect words with print.
- **Writing words** – note that the ability to write whole words including their names is an eventual learning goal, with many children doing this only at the end of the reception year. This is because children need to develop a 'visual' memory of what symbols they need and this usually happens as children learn to read.

Delivering this aspect of learning

As with reading, some parents will need reassurance that by encouraging children's mark making or 'scribbling', children are actually learning about writing. The need for children to 'write' by themselves and gain confidence in expressing themselves is paramount. Most children will write when they are playing and feel that their writing is not being judged.

Good practice checklist

- Is there a 'writing' area with a range of interesting materials for children to use?
- Are name cards and letters present on the writing table?
- Do children see adults writing in the setting?
- Are writing materials provided alongside the role-play area, e.g. pencil and pad by the toy telephone?
- Do adults and children regularly make up stories, which the adult writes down?
- Are opportunities created for 'real' writing, e.g. 'Would you like to sign this birthday card for Jake?'
- Is there a message or display board for children to pin up their writing?

Handwriting

This aspect looks primarily at the physical skills that need to be developed in order that children can later produce fluent handwriting. It is increasingly being recognised that young children's physical development cannot be 'fast tracked' and the gross motor movements need to be in place before we can expect children to make accurate small movements.

Key messages in the Stepping Stones and Early Learning Goals

◆ **Hand-eye co-ordination and use of one-handed tools and equipment** – the first Stepping Stone is not linked to pencil or actual writing. The aim of this Stepping Stone is to develop children's hands and overall co-ordination.

◆ **Gross motor movement** – is a key step in children's later ability to write. Children who have not made large writing movements and skip this step are likely to develop poor writing posture and grip.

◆ **Form recognisable letters** – is a later Stepping Stone, with most children achieving good pencil control and correctly formed letters at the end of the reception year. This means that tracing and traditional types of teaching of letter formation are not suitable for children on the other Stepping Stones.

Delivering this aspect of learning

This is another aspect of learning which some parents become concerned about. Make sure that they see the importance of developing children's hand and general co-ordination before putting pressure on children to actually 'write'.

In terms of helping children to write, it is important that large gross movements are regularly promoted and that children get the opportunity to make marks on a large scale frequently.

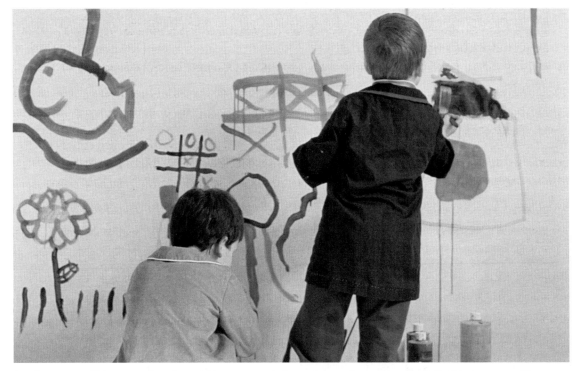

Are there areas within your setting where children can use chalk or paint on a large scale, e.g. plastic sheeting on a wall?

Good practice checklist

◆ Are there areas within your setting where children can use chalk or paint on a large scale, e.g. plastic sheeting on a wall?

◆ Are activities regularly provided that will encourage a range of hand movements, e.g. pinching, twisting, turning?

◆ Do you regularly use ribbons or scarves to encourage children to make large circular or vertical movements in the air?

◆ Are games played with children that will promote fine motor skills, e.g. spooning rice into bottles or playing pick up sticks?

Specific activities for promoting communication, language and literacy

Many of the Stepping Stones and Early Learning Goals for this area of learning can be promoted through activities that can be adapted to suit the theme

One-to-one adult support and attention

Many settings will need to look at their routine to find ways of allowing children time either in very small groups or, preferably, gaining one-to-one support from an adult. This time needs to be spent in encouraging children to talk, to express their ideas, and also to enjoy listening to stories. This may be achieved by placing an adult in the book area so that children can 'drop by' when they feel like it.

Modelling language

Children need to have language modelled so that they can at first absorb it and subsequently use it. We can do this in two key ways.

1 Adults can 'narrate' as they are working with children, e.g. 'I am not sure that this is going to be *effective*, it may not work.'
2 Puppets and cuddly toys can be brought in to act as stooges, e.g. 'I'll ask teddy what he thinks …'

Creating writing opportunities

Find 'real' reasons why children may wish to write, put writing materials in the role-play area, ask children to sign cards, write letters and make their own labels. Puppets and cuddly toys can also be the cue to write as they may ask the children to jot things down for them.

Rhymes

There are many rhyme books available. Planning a programme of teaching rhymes is important so that children can build up a good repertoire.

Look out for any of these:

◆ *Round and Round the Garden: Play Rhymes for Young Children*
◆ *The Collins Book of Nursery Rhymes*
◆ *Rub a dub dub: Favourite nursery rhymes*
◆ *The Oxford Nursery Book*

Valuing communication, language and literacy

It is essential that we resist any temptation to 'fast track' children through this area of learning. Handwriting in particular is linked to children's physical development and research shows that children who have been pushed to write 'small' letters are less likely to have fluent handwriting later on. Equally, children who have become frustrated by being pushed to decode words before they have developed their auditory and visual discrimination are less likely to read for pleasure.

- ◆ Videotape or photograph children as they are 'mark making' or 'play writing' so that parents can see how much effort they are making.
- ◆ Assess children's fine motor development accurately, e.g. can children pour out a drink without spilling it, can they squeeze a sponge repeatedly?
- ◆ Share children's particular interest in books with parents.
- ◆ Make sure parents know which nursery rhymes are being learned and how this will help children to hear sounds and patterns in words.
- ◆ Ask children to 'explain' their thoughts to see how their language for thinking is developing.
- ◆ Make sure children's attempts to write are greeted with interest and wherever possible write back to children – writing is about communication, not about letter formation.
- ◆ Encourage parents to be good role models by writing and reading in front of their children.

Activity – Communication, language and literacy
Rhymes and songs are a key way in which children can learn about language and rhymes.
    Produce a pack that contains the words and some props for three well-known nursery rhymes or songs.

Mathematical development

This is an important area of learning, as children need to have experienced mathematics in a practical way before formal recording.
    There are three aspects of learning.

Aspects of learning	Curriculum guidance page
Numbers as labels and for counting	74
Calculating	76
Shape, space and measures	78–80

Numbers as labels and for counting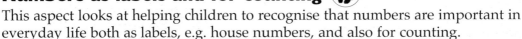

This aspect looks at helping children to recognise that numbers are important in everyday life both as labels, e.g. house numbers, and also for counting.

Key messages in the Stepping Stones and Early Learning Goals

- ◆ **Using the names of numbers** – the starting point in the first Stepping Stone is that children should know a few of the names of numbers without necessarily understanding how many '2' is. The ability to recognise some numbers is a later Stepping Stone with the knowledge of numbers from one to nine an Early Learning Goal for most children at the end of their reception year.

◆ **Counting** – at first children will 'pretend' to count rather than matching a number to each object systematically. The ability for children to match three or four objects to numbers as they count is a later Stepping Stone, which most children will be ready to achieve at the start of their reception year.

Delivering this aspect of learning

The starting point for children is to learn the language of number. This needs to be modelled by practitioners as frequently as possible, e.g. 'There are six of you wanting to play.' In order for children to start recognising written numerals, they will need to experience them in the environment. You can use cards with numbers on them to put next to groups of objects, e.g. a table with three chairs may have a '3' put on top of it. Number rhymes and songs will also help children to learn the 'labels' of numbers.

Once children have begun to recognise numbers, especially those that are important to them such as their age, they may begin to try to write them. Children will also need to see adults counting and be put in situations where counting seems natural, e.g. 'How many steps – shall we count them?'

Good practice checklist

◆ Are number rhymes and songs included in the planning?
◆ Are numerals displayed in context, e.g. a notice saying 'Five children can play here'?
◆ How are everyday opportunities to count included in the routine, e.g. 'How many children want to have a snack now? Let's count?'
◆ Are activities regularly planned that encourage children to sort objects?
◆ Do role-play areas give opportunities for children to use number, e.g. Chinese takeaway, coins in a till?
◆ Are simple board games that involve counting regularly played?
◆ Are physical games and activities planned which involve counting, e.g. 'What's the time, Mr Wolf?'

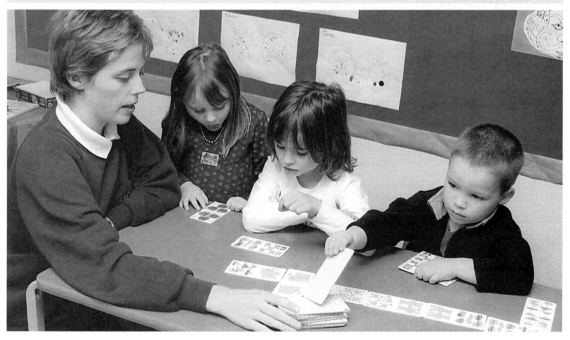

Are simple games that involve counting regularly played?

- ◆ Do adults regularly write down numerals for children, e.g. 'You have two paintings to take home, I will write two on my pad to help me remember'?
- ◆ Do adults point to objects or items as they are counting them?
- ◆ Are opportunities such as birthdays maximised to help children see and recognise numbers, e.g. candles on a cake, displays of children who are three, four and five years old?

Calculating

This aspect of learning is not about formal 'sums' but about helping children to solve problems in a mathematical way.

Key messages in the Stepping Stones and Early Learning Goals

- ◆ **Grouping and comparing objects** – is a recurring theme in the Stepping Stones because by comparing and grouping objects children can see the differences between them, e.g. 'this group has more' or 'together there are …'
- ◆ **Language** – is a major feature of this aspect of learning as children will need to know how to express what they are thinking.

Delivering this aspect of learning

It is important to recognise that this aspect of learning is not about writing or doing 'sums'. This may need to be explained to parents and adults who are unfamiliar with the Foundation Stage. The key to delivering this aspect of learning is to provide practical experiences of comparing and bringing together groups of objects. Children will also need to hear the language of calculating modelled for them, e.g. 'this one has the most' or 'this one has two more'. There should also be scope in everyday routines for children to see 'maths in action', e.g. 'Are there enough pieces of apple for everyone?'

Good practice checklist

- ◆ Do adults, including parents, understand that formal recording of number is not required?
- ◆ Are opportunities planned for children to group and sort objects?
- ◆ Are adults setting up problems for children to solve, e.g. 'Is there enough to go around?'
- ◆ Are games planned that involve adding or taking away objects, e.g. roll a dice, take the number of buttons shown, who has got the most?
- ◆ Are everyday routines used to encourage children to add and take away, e.g. 'We have too many chairs. Can you take one away? How many are left now?'

Shape, space and measures

This aspect of learning helps children to learn practically about three concepts: shape, space and measures. It is important that children experience all three in practical terms as this knowledge will be built on when they begin more formal mathematics.

Key messages in the Stepping Stones and Early Learning Goals

- ◆ **Using shapes** – is recurrent in all of the Stepping Stones. Children need to use and handle shapes practically, e.g. in construction activities. They also need to learn to recognise and label shapes.
- ◆ **Positional and other mathematical language** – is required for children to be able to explain and develop their thinking, e.g. 'shorter', 'heavier', 'in front of', 'inside'.

◆ **Ordering and comparing** – comes in the last Stepping Stone, although some children will naturally begin to notice differences between the lengths and sizes of objects. Note that the last Stepping Stone suggests children will need practice at ordering two objects by height or length.

Delivering this aspect of learning

This is a very practical aspect of learning. Children need activities that encourage them to touch and handle shapes. Encourage them to use construction equipment as well as boxes and other shapes. Language plays an essential part: by hearing positional and other language children's thinking can be extended. Problem solving with a puppet or other stooge may be useful here, e.g. 'Teddy has six buttons – which box will they fit in – the largest or the smallest box?'

Children are naturally good at comparing – they quickly notice, for example, if someone has a larger drink or a bigger biscuit. Working with children's natural curiosity to compare is therefore important. Activities such as measuring which container holds the most water will help children to learn about capacity as well as ordering.

Note that formal teaching of time or measurements is not required – the key is to make sure that children are gaining practical mathematical experience.

Good practice checklist

◆ Is construction play regularly planned into a session?
◆ Do adults set children challenges, e.g. 'Can you make the train track into a circle?'
◆ Are activities regularly planned for children to weigh and compare objects?
◆ Are activities planned which encourage children to use 2D and 3D shapes, e.g. squares, circles of paper?
◆ Are children encouraged to look out for shapes in their environment, e.g. panes of glass, shapes of doors?
◆ Are activities planned that help children to order and to sort according to size, weight or shape?
◆ Are games played where positional language is used, e.g. hide and seek and treasure hunts with children giving each other instructions?

Specific activities for promoting mathematical development

There is a range of adaptable activities that can be used to help children's mathematical development.

Sorting objects

By playing sorting games with objects that are interesting to them, children tend naturally to compare, count and notice the differences between objects. Large trays are useful for children to sort on, as they are able to put objects into different corners or piles, e.g. they may decide to sort buttons into colours. Sensitive adult intervention is then important to extend children's mathematical thinking – 'Which pile has the most buttons?'

Everyday routines

Children should be encouraged to pour drinks, put out cups, beakers and plates as part of an everyday routine. This needs to be accompanied by some adult narrative and even some gentle questioning if appropriate, e.g. 'How many cups have we got so far? Let's count to check there are enough.'

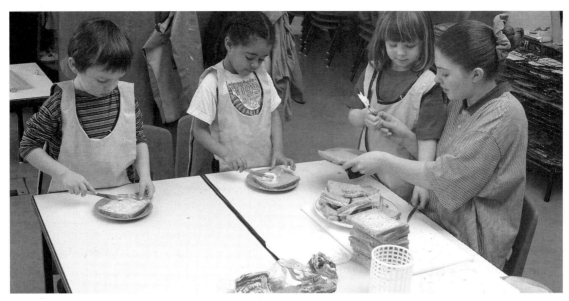

Children should be encouraged to pour drinks, put out cups, beakers and plates as part of an everyday routine

Using puppets and stooges
As with other areas of learning, this provides a key way in which adults can set children challenges, but also model language. 'Teddy is trying to build up a house of bricks – he wants to know where he should put this one. He thinks it should go inside, but what do you think?'

Physical activities
Combining physical activities with this area of learning can help children to 'physically' feel numbers and experience shape, space and measures. Children can roll a dice and then step or jump according to the number shown. Other games such as 'How many steps can you take with this shell on the spoon?' will help children to measure as well as count. Outdoor activities can also include number treasure hunts, where children have to find objects hidden in the outdoor area and, if they are developmentally ready, match them to the correct numeral.

Valuing mathematical development
Mathematics is one area of the curriculum in which adults often feel insecure. Parents and even practitioners may have had poor experiences of mathematics at school. This can lead to adults concentrating more on the 'answers' than on seeing that children are gaining confidence and enjoying the process.

Good practice checklist
◆ Make sure parents understand that children will be doing mathematics, even if it is not being formally recorded.
◆ Put up displays that show how mathematics is being done, e.g. 'Today Anne and Raj looked at these leaves. This one is the biggest leaf. This one is the smallest leaf. Altogether there are six leaves.'
◆ Make sure activities are fun and that children do not feel pressurised to get the 'right' answer.

◆ Remember that formal recording of numerals is not necessary as children should be learning practically.

◆ Encourage mathematical experiences in the role-play area, e.g. putting out the balancing scales in a shop.

◆ Encourage children to guess and predict – these are important mathematical skills that need building.

Activity – Mathematical development

Children can learn about number through many everyday activities.

Choose one everyday activity, which forms part of the routine of your work setting, about which to write an activity plan.

Your activity plan should show:

◆ how the activity links to the Stepping Stones or Early Learning Goals in mathematical development;

◆ the role of the adult during the activity.

Knowledge and understanding of the world

This area is full of surprises, with the emphasis firmly on children's experiences and their world. It should help them to reflect on their environment and to learn from it. It is important that each of the aspects is carefully read. Many topics and activities commonly used by some settings will no longer be relevant to this area of learning.

There are six aspects of learning.

Aspects of learning	Curriculum guidance page
Exploration and investigation	86, 88
Designing and making skills	90
Information and communication technology	92
Sense of time	94
Sense of place	96
Cultures and beliefs	98

Exploration and investigation

This aspect encourages children to touch, feel and observe a variety of objects and materials.

Key messages in the Stepping Stones and Early Learning Goals

◆ **Curiosity** – is one main focus that runs through the Stepping Stones. If children are presented with interesting materials and resources, they will want to discuss, explore and therefore identify features of objects.

◆ **Sorting and patterns** – this may come as a surprise to some practitioners as sorting, noticing and making patterns is often associated with mathematics.

◆ **Noticing change** – in the first Stepping Stone this is about children being interested in how things work. Later on, children should be questioning and trying to work out how things have changed and why.

Delivering this aspect of learning

This is a wonderful aspect of learning to deliver: it is very wide and open. Children need a selection of interesting resources, artefacts and objects to observe, handle and sort. The development of children's language is also key as they need to learn how to phrase questions and develop sufficient vocabulary to talk about what is happening.

> ### Good practice checklist
> ◆ Is a range of materials suitable for sorting available, e.g. buttons, shells, old and new toys, and cards?
> ◆ Are resources such as magnifying glasses and bug boxes available to encourage children to observe closely?
> ◆ Do adults draw children's notice to particular features of objects?
> ◆ Are there opportunities for children to plant and grow things?
> ◆ Are activities provided that will help children observe changes, e.g. ice cubes in the water tray, cooking activities?
> ◆ Are there collections of objects such as pepper grinders and kaleidoscopes that can be safely taken apart for children to understand how they work?

Designing and making skills

This aspect of learning looks at developing children's ability to use tools and make things. It links closely to aspects within creative development, physical development and mathematical development.

Key messages in the Stepping Stones and Early Learning Goals

◆ **Construction** – in the first Stepping Stone, children are to be encouraged to use construction kits and toys, as well as being introduced to materials such as paper and card, and modelling materials such as dough and clay. Eventually, the aim is for children to choose materials to make items of their own design.

◆ **Selecting tools** – the aim is that children should understand what different tools can do as well as being able to use them safely.

Delivering this aspect of learning

The guidance for practitioners suggests that children need specific adult input so that they learn how to use tools safely and properly. The guidance also outlines the types of tools that children might use. These include staplers and junior hacksaws as well as more mundane items such as glue spreaders and scissors. The guidance is clear that children should be designing for themselves, so very adult-directed activities that do not encourage children to problem-solve, choose and design will not cover this aspect of learning.

> ### Good practice checklist
> ◆ Has the setting a good range of tools and materials?
> ◆ Are adults able to provide guidance for children as to how to construct things, e.g. learning how to fold paper, using a stapler?
> ◆ Are cooking activities regularly carried out that allow children to 'experiment' in some way, e.g. deciding which type of topping to have or what to include in a salad?
> ◆ Are 'problems' given to children, e.g. 'Teddy would like a new hat – can you make one?'
> ◆ Are children supported, but not directed, by adults when they make items?
> ◆ Do adults model the language children need to talk about their work?

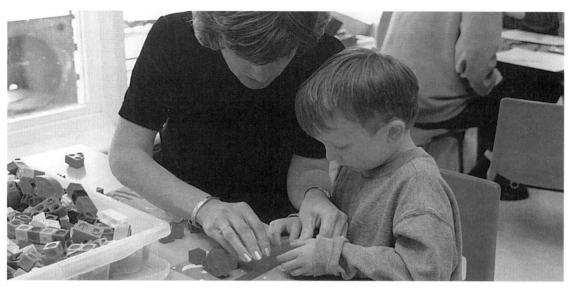

Are adults able to provide guidance for children as to how to construct things, e.g. learning how to fold paper, using a stapler?

Information and communication technology

As an aspect in its own right, it is essential it is not overlooked. The guidance does not suggest that very young children will necessarily need to use a computer, but resources necessary to deliver this aspect will be required by the setting.

Key messages in the Stepping Stones and Early Learning Goals
◆ **Operate equipment** – the focus of the first Stepping Stone is to encourage children to be interested in using ICT such as remote-controlled cars. The later Stepping Stones expect that they can use a simple computer programme.

Delivering this aspect of learning
The starting point for this aspect of learning is to make sure that your setting has a wide range of resources available for the children to use. The guidance suggests remote-controlled cars, tape recorders, radios and videos, as well as computers. It is important that young children are active in their learning, so using equipment where they can see 'cause and effect' is useful.

> ### Good practice checklist
> ◆ Is there a range of equipment for children to use?
> ◆ Are adults in the setting comfortable about their own ICT knowledge?
> ◆ Is software suitable for age/stage of children?
> ◆ Are tape recorders used in the setting and can children operate them, e.g. to hear a story, to record messages?
> ◆ Are 'cause and effect' toys available for children to play with, e.g. remote-controlled cars, roamer turtles?

Sense of time

This aspect of learning will help children understand the concept of time. Note that this aspect does not refer to the teaching of time, but time in terms of events in children's lives and those of their families and people they know. In the long term, this aspect of learning links to history, although the key is to stimulate children's interest.

Key messages in the Stepping Stones and Early Learning Goals

◆ **Significant events** – this is the key to the Stepping Stones and the Early Learning Goal. At first, children need just to talk about what has happened in their lives. Eventually, the aim is that children can understand past and present as well as old and new.

◆ **Find out about past and present** – this is the Early Learning Goal, with children being able to ask questions and look at source material such as old toys or photographs.

Delivering this aspect of learning

The key to delivering this aspect is to find time to listen and to talk to children. This is crucial, as each child will have very different memories and experiences that need to be drawn on. You also need to make sure that events that are important to children are followed up, e.g. after a visit to a farm, it is important to encourage children to talk about what they remember.

Children also need to have access to resources that will trigger memories and discussion.

> ### Good practice checklist
> ◆ Are children regularly having time to talk in pairs or on a one-to-one basis with adults?
> ◆ Are activities planned that will help children learn the language they need to describe events that have happened in the past?
> ◆ Are objects brought into the setting that encourage children's curiosity about the past?
> ◆ Are activities planned that will help children's sequencing skills, e.g. photos of themselves as babies, toddlers and now?
> ◆ Are memorable activities planned that will help children talk about what they have done, e.g. visits to a local park?

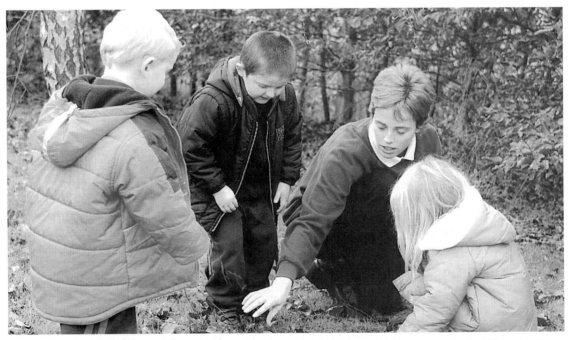

Are memorable activities planned that will help children talk about what they have done, e.g. visits to a local park?

Sense of place

This aspect concentrates on children's experiences of their local environment.

Key messages in the Stepping Stones and Early Learning Goals

- **Interest in where they live** – is in the first Stepping Stone. If children are able to observe and take an interest in their local environment, they will eventually be able to compare and identify particular features of environments.
- **Observe** – this is a key way in which children are expected to find out about their environments. The aim is to make sure that children can learn about their environment in a practical rather than abstract way.

Delivering this aspect of learning

It is important to understand that this aspect of learning is not to do with environments outside the child's knowledge. Topics such as 'seaside' or 'farms' will only be relevant if children have actually experienced these places. This represents a significant shift of emphasis. It is important to plan walks and trips so that children can visit and think about their local area. If this is not possible, consider taking photographs or videos of places you know children visit regularly, e.g. park, swimming pool, supermarket.

> ### Good practice checklist
>
> - Are parents being involved in this aspect of learning, e.g. looking out for things on the way home with their child?
> - Are trips regularly organised in the local vicinity?
> - Is the outdoor area being used to encourage children to notice differences?
> - Are maps incorporated into children's play, e.g. a street map in the role-play area or an atlas in the story area?
> - Do adults in the setting model the language that children will need, e.g. 'countryside', 'town', 'park', 'village', 'house'?
> - Are photographs of environments similar to ones in the children's experience available?

Cultures and beliefs

The aim of this aspect of learning is to help children learn about their own as well as other's beliefs. This is seen as a very gradual process, beginning with children learning and thinking about their own feelings. This represents a marked shift of emphasis as many early years settings had been encouraged to get young children to find out about cultures other than their own. This is no longer an appropriate approach for most children until they reach the reception year. This aspect of learning should be looked at with 'sense of community' in the 'Personal, social and emotional development' area of learning.

Key messages in the Stepping Stones and Early Learning Goals

- **Significant events** – the starting point for this aspect of learning. Children need to think about things that are important to them and their family members. This might be birthdays, weddings, funerals, as well as holidays and days out.
- **Awareness of others cultures and beliefs** – is a green Stepping Stone, which suggests that most children will be ready to look at this in the reception year.

It would still be advisable to choose cultures and beliefs that are represented in the community if possible.

Delivering this aspect of learning

This aspect of learning requires that we spend time listening to children and their families so that we can develop their sense of identity. This is particularly important in situations where children are not feeling confident about who they are. Look for opportunities to celebrate special moments in their lives with children, however trivial they may appear, e.g. getting a new pair of shoes or going to a friend's for tea. By helping them to see the importance of events in their lives, they will gain self-awareness.

Good practice checklist

- ◆ Do adults spend time on a one-to-one basis with children in the setting?
- ◆ Are displays regularly used that encourage children to talk about special moments in their lives?
- ◆ Do adults listen carefully to children in sustained conversations?
- ◆ Are naturally occurring opportunities to make children aware of different cultures and beliefs taken, e.g. noticing the way in which people dress in photographs or images?
- ◆ Are positive views of other cultures being shown to children rather than 'tourist' views, e.g. most people living in Hawaii do not wear grass skirts?

Specific activities for promoting knowledge and understanding of the world

This area of learning has some diverse elements. This means that several different types of activities should be planned for.

Sorting activities

You will need to provide regular opportunities for children to sort through materials, resources and items. The best types of items to choose for sorting activities should allow children various possibilities, e.g. size, colour, shape, texture.

Designing and making activities

Look for opportunities for children to make items that can then be used as part of the role-play area, e.g. dough cakes for the bakers or toys for the toy shop (see pp. 216, 233).

Puppets and cuddly toys

Puppets and cuddly toys not only provide a good way of modelling language to children, they can also be the reason why children may wish to make things, e.g. 'Teddy wants a cupboard to keep his honey pots in.'

Tape recorders, hand-held vacuum cleaners, etc

Encourage children to use story tapes and to be responsible for turning tape recorders on and off. Consider buying a hand-held vacuum cleaner, preferably battery operated, as this will allow children to hoover areas, e.g. clear up sand, while helping them to understand how equipment works.

Valuing Knowledge and understanding of the world

It is important for parents to understand that this area of learning is very much based around children's own worlds and that it provides the foundation for the later disciplines of history, geography and science. Consider taking photographs of children exploring the outside area, or going on a walk and labelling the skills that the children are learning from this. It is also important that parents understand IT skills do not have to begin with an actual computer and that children will gain by learning about the broad range of technology.

Activity – *Knowledge and understanding of the world*

Much of the emphasis in this area of learning is based on children's own experiences of the world.

Using photographs taken during a week in the work setting, help a group of children to produce a simple book.

Evaluate this activity and consider how it links to the Stepping Stones and Early Learning Goals within 'Knowledge and understanding of the world'.

Physical development

The importance of physical development is increasingly recognised not only for children's health, but also in terms of their cognitive development. This area of learning covers children's gross and fine motor skills and also their ability to use tools and awareness of how to keep healthy.

There are five aspects of learning.

Aspects of learning	Curriculum guidance page
Sense of space	104
Movement	106, 108
Health and bodily awareness	110
Using equipment	112
Using tools and materials	114

Sense of space

This aspect of learning is about children enjoying space and developing some spatial awareness.

Key messages in the Stepping Stones and Early Learning Goals

- **Rhythm and music** – is in the first Stepping Stone and can be delivered by putting on music or encouraging children to explore and move with musical instruments. In the later Stepping Stones, they are expected to use movement and gesture to show feelings.
- **Movement in a range of ways** – comes in all of the Stepping Stones. Children should be encouraged to jump, skip, hop, slide, run, etc. They should also be learning how to stop and control their movements.

Delivering this aspect of learning

Children will need access to space in or out of doors, preferably both. You will also need to provide a range of equipment that will encourage children to make a variety of movements, e.g. something to jump off or climb on. It is important for adults to be aware of safety issues, while not imposing too many rules which will prevent children from exploring and enjoying their movements. Adults will also need to help children learn language associated with movement and space. This can be done through games but also by gently commenting on what children are doing, e.g. 'You twisted and jumped.'

Good practice checklist

◆ Are there regular times each day or session when children have access to space?
◆ Is a range of equipment provided that will encourage children to make different movements?
◆ Are games planned, which encourage children to stop, freeze or copy a movement?
◆ Do you have a range of music tapes and instruments that will encourage children to move to a rhythm?
◆ Are adults modelling language of movement with children, e.g. 'follow, lead, slide'?
◆ Are children aware of the boundaries so that they can keep safe?

Movement

This aspect of learning looks at developing children's fine and gross movements. It also links closely to children's sense of space, so both aspects of learning need to be looked at together.

Key messages in the Stepping Stones and Early Learning Goals

◆ **Using various parts of the body** – this looks at developing balance and movements that will strengthen and develop co-ordination, e.g. squatting, kneeling and climbing.
◆ **Manipulate materials** – this is in the green Stepping Stone on p. 106 of Curriculum guidance, although many children will be manipulating small objects before this.
◆ **Judge space and body position** – children should increasingly be aware of how much space they need and be aware of others. This is linked to their perceptual skills.

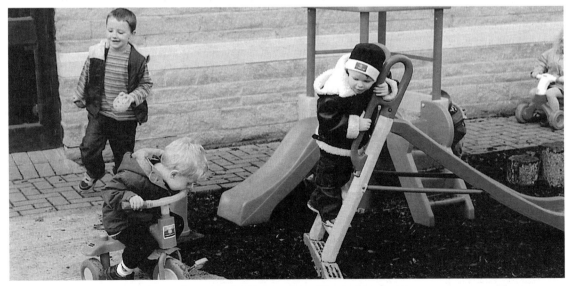

Is a range of equipment provided that will encourage children to make different movements?

Delivering this aspect of learning

The starting point must be looking carefully at children's physical development and confidence. For example, some children will be able to run on tiptoe in and out of objects while others find it hard to move around safely.

Good practice checklist

- Are there any areas in your setting where children can 'squeeze' in and hide so that they can be aware of small spaces?
- Are activities provided that encourage children to find pairs, make circles?
- Do you play games such as 'follow my leader' with children?
- Are activities provided that encourage children to make repeated small movements, e.g. picking out blue rice grains from a tray of red rice?
- Are boundaries marked out so that children understand the spaces in which certain play activities should be kept, e.g. a chalk line around the role-play area so that they keep pushchairs within it?
- Are children encouraged to make their own small spaces, e.g. dens, cardboard-box cars?

Health and bodily awareness

This aspect of learning is about helping children to understand how to keep healthy and to have an awareness of their bodies.

Key messages in the Stepping Stones and Early Learning Goals

- **Healthy practices** – the first Stepping Stone is about helping children to recognise their needs and to talk about them. This leads to children being able to make links, e.g. between hygiene and not becoming ill. Note that activities to make children aware of keeping healthy are to be introduced as children get older, e.g. in the green Stepping Stone and as an Early Learning Goal.
- **Changes to their bodies** – the idea behind this is that children gradually learn to associate feeling hot or tired with changes to their bodies and understand how this happens. Note that this strand is not mentioned in the first Stepping Stone.

Delivering this aspect of learning

This aspect of learning needs careful planning and thought. The aim is not to condemn families' lifestyles or approaches to food! The focus is on helping children become aware that there is a connection between their bodies and diet, hygiene and exercise. Much of this aspect of learning needs to be delivered by helping them to make connections for themselves and by good role modelling by adults in the setting.

Good practice checklist

- Is water provided for children to drink after they have been exercising?
- Are fruit and vegetables provided for children as snacks?
- Do adults talk to children about the temperature and weather and the type of clothing that is needed?
- Are children given the reasons for hygiene practices, e.g. 'When we wash our hands, we wash away all the germs that otherwise we may eat'?
- Do children have easy access to paper tissues to wipe their noses?
- Are hand washing and toileting facilities pleasant for children to use, e.g. attractive soaps, paper towels, warm water?
- Do adults in the setting demonstrate positive attitudes towards going outdoors and taking exercise?

Using equipment

This aspect of learning has links with the next aspect of learning, 'Using tools and materials'. The type of equipment that is specifically mentioned in the guidance includes beanbags, balls, tricycles and small world toys (such as playmobil, train sets).

Key messages in the Stepping Stones and Early Learning Goals

◆ **Control** – is emphasised throughout the Stepping Stones. The aim is that children should learn how to control and use equipment. This means that children will often need to practise particular movements. Pushing and pulling, for example, is stated in the first Stepping Stone.

◆ **Throwing and catching** – is in the green Stepping Stone and is of particular importance because it benefits many areas of development, especially cognitive development.

Delivering this aspect of learning

This aspect of learning looks particularly at the type of equipment that is common in most early years settings, e.g. tricycles, large wheeled apparatus, objects for throwing and catching, as well as equipment that might be found in small world areas, e.g. train set with points.

> ### Good practice checklist
>
> ◆ Is equipment appropriate for children's stage of development, e.g. tricycles of the right size and that can take the weight?
> ◆ Are activities planned to develop children's catching and throwing skills?
> ◆ Are children given sufficient time to 'master' equipment, e.g. enough time to learn to control and steer the tricycle?
> ◆ Are children encouraged to vary the equipment they usually play with?

Using tools and materials

This aspect centres especially on developing children's hand-eye co-ordination and fine motor skills in relation to tools.

Key messages in the Stepping Stones and Early Learning Goals

◆ **Hand-eye activities** – this is an important starting point for children to be able to use tools, hence its position in the first Stepping Stone. It may include cooking activities, pouring and scooping in sand and water trays.

◆ **One-handed tools and equipment** – is in the first Stepping Stone. The aim is that children begin to use equipment such as scissors, pencils, paintbrushes, etc. The later Stepping Stones look at children becoming more skilled in their use.

◆ **Safety** – looks at the need for children to understand how to use tools safely. The green Stepping Stone suggests that children should have enough understanding to be able to use some tools without the need for direct supervision.

Delivering this aspect of learning

The starting point for this aspect of learning is to make sure that a range of activities is provided that will encourage children to use hand-eye co-ordination. Children also need to be provided with a range of tools so that they can learn to manipulate them.

Good practice checklist

◆ Are tools and materials attractive?
◆ Do adults give children the reasons behind any of the 'safety' rules?
◆ Is a range of scissors provided for different purposes, e.g. left handed, zig-zag, sharp enough to cut fabric?
◆ Are children encouraged to choose tools themselves?
◆ Are materials provided that will encourage children to explore, e.g. dough, malleable materials, clay?
◆ Are adults able to give support to children rather than take over the use of a tool?

Specific activities for promoting physical development

Many of the Stepping Stones and Early Learning Goals for this area of learning can be delivered by adapting some basic activities.

Obstacle courses

Obstacle courses will help children to learn naturally about movement and space. They can be planned as indoor as well as outdoor activities, e.g. cushions put on a floor for children to avoid. Children can be encouraged to use equipment with them, e.g. take a pram for a walk or follow an obstacle course on a tricycle.

Sand, water, dough and paint

These core activities will encourage children to use their hand-eye co-ordination. Equipment such as funnels, scoops and beakers, should also be provided so that they learn to manipulate them.

Designing and making projects

Children need to learn that tools have a purpose. Activities that help them to design and make things will help them to practise using tools such as scissors or staplers. Activities could include making clothes for a favourite cuddly toy, turning a box into a car to sit in, or making a card for a favourite person.

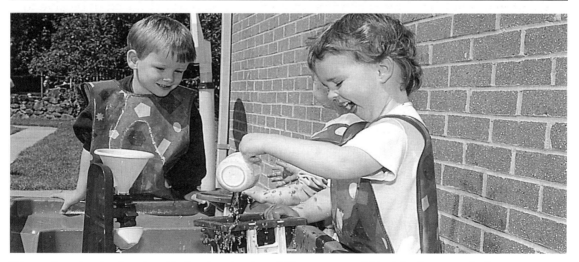

Using equipment such as funnels and beakers in water play activities encourages children's hand-eye co-ordination

Valuing physical development

Parents do not always see the importance of physical development in children's overall development. It is important to explain to parents that by building children's physical skills they will be more co-ordinated for other activities such as writing. There is a growing body of evidence that links brain development to physical development.

Good practice checklist

◆ Take photographs of children engaged in physical play – add captions, which explain the learning benefits, e.g. social interaction, visual discrimination, spatial awareness.

Activity – Physical development

Make a simple obstacle course for children, which will help to promote their gross and locomotive skills.

Evaluate this activity in terms of how it covers the Stepping Stones and Early Learning Goals for this area of learning. Consider ways in which children could be involved in the future design and making of obstacle courses.

Creative development

Creative development encompasses a wide range of experiences that we should provide for children. These include poetry, dance, music, as well as a range of materials to model and mark make with.

There are four aspects of learning.

Aspects of learning	Curriculum guidance page
Exploring media and materials	120
Music	122
Imagination	124
Responding to experiences, and expressing and communicating ideas	126

Exploring media and materials

This is a wide aspect of learning, which covers children's awareness of colour, texture and structures.

Key messages in the Stepping Stones and Early Learning Goals

◆ **Colour** – is one of the points of emphasis in this aspect. At first children should be differentiating between colours with the eventual aim that they should be able to choose colours for particular purposes and know what happens when colours are mixed.

◆ **Texture** – this comes in all of the Stepping Stones. Children should be given access to various textures and learn how to describe texture. The aim is that they should be able to create different textures. Adults need to talk to children about different textures.

◆ **Structures** – as a first step towards modelling, children should have opportunities to build different types of structures. These could be using boxes or bricks, as well as junk modelling.

Delivering this aspect of learning

The aim of this aspect of learning is to encourage children to become aware of colour, texture and structures, and to explore for themselves what each can do. You need to make sure children are given a range of materials to work with and that they have sufficient time and confidence to experiment and see what they can do. The focus of creative development is for children to experiment rather than necessarily produce perfect products. It is also worth noting that the green Stepping Stone suggests that they need to be able to work on a large and a small scale.

Good practice checklist

- Are children encouraged to mix colours when painting?
- Do adults in the setting talk about the colours that children are producing and 'label' them?
- Do children have access to a wide range of painting materials including brushes, sponges and printing blocks, as well as rollers?
- Are children able to paint on a large as well as a small scale?
- Are children able to use a range of mark making materials including chalks, pastels and charcoals, as well as felt tips and markers?
- Are children given opportunities to play with malleable materials and to model with them?
- Does your setting have a wide range of interesting materials for children to use, e.g. ribbons, laces, wool, card, boxes, different types of paper?
- Are children encouraged to choose their own materials?
- Do adults in the setting understand that their role should be a supporting rather than a directing one?
- Is praise and encouragement directed at the process of 'creating' or only for end products?
- Are children encouraged to look at what other children are making and designing?
- Are adults in the setting showing children how to use particular techniques, e.g. how to join materials, as a way of supporting them?

Music

This aspect of learning looks at helping children to respond to music and to use musical instruments.

Key messages in the Stepping Stones and Early Learning Goals

- **Songs** – this is a strong strand within this aspect. Children are expected to join in and have favourite songs that eventually they know by heart. In the blue Stepping Stone children are encouraged to make up their own songs.
- **Making music** – this begins with children exploring instruments, but as they move through the Stepping Stones they should be able to see how to alter the sound they make, e.g. loud and soft or higher and lower notes.
- **Movement to music** – at first, children need to just move their bodies or hands in response to sounds. This should become more controlled with children being able to move rhythmically by, for example, moving to the beat.

Delivering this aspect of learning

Many settings are good at singing songs with children, although some find it harder to get out the musical instruments. If instruments are not available to children, they

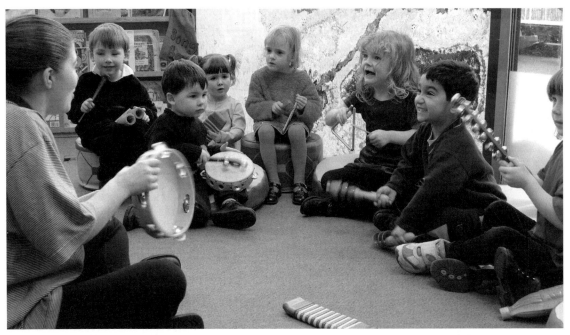

Are instruments put out regularly for children to use?

are unable to make progress and develop ways of using them effectively. It is important for children to listen to music with strong beats so that they can hear them easily.

> ### Good practice checklist
> ◆ Are instruments put out regularly for children to use?
> ◆ Are children encouraged to try and make loud, soft, fast and slow sounds with instruments?
> ◆ Are clapping games and songs used with children?
> ◆ Are children encouraged to make up their own songs?
> ◆ Are songs with actions or for children to dance to regularly planned, e.g. 'Okey hokey', 'Farmer in the den', 'In and out the dusty bluebells'?
> ◆ Is music played that will help children to move to the beat?

Imagination

This aspect of learning looks at encouraging children to imagine and to help them to use their imagination in art, dance, drama and role play.

Key messages in the Stepping Stones and Early Learning Goals
◆ **Role play** – this runs throughout this aspect with children at first repeating movements and actions that they have seen. Role play is expected to develop and become more sophisticated with children acting out scenarios and stories that they have made up.
◆ **Stories** – the aim of including stories in this aspect is to help children recreate story lines into their play. They may, for example, draw a picture and narrate it based on a story that they have heard or thought of.

Delivering this aspect of learning

The key to delivering this aspect of learning is to make sure children have access to plenty of props, small world toys and dressing-up materials. This will help them to create their own worlds. Children can also enjoy recreating a story, especially if props have been used during the telling of it. Pretend play is also linked to children's language development. This means that we need to look for ways of developing their vocabulary and speech – this is why reading stories to them will be of benefit, as by hearing new language in context it becomes easier to repeat.

Good practice checklist

- Is there a good range of clean, exciting props for children to use?
- Is the role-play area interesting and slightly hidden from view?
- Are activities involving story bags regularly planned?
- Are children given access to story bags so that they can recreate the story?
- Do adults 'play' with children when invited to do so?
- Are opportunities taken to use the role-play area as a backdrop for well-known stories, e.g. three bears' house?
- Are children given enough time to develop their own pretend play?
- Are stories chosen that will allow children to re-create them?

Responding to experiences, and expressing and communicating ideas

This is a wide aspect of learning and in some ways an accumulation of the other aspects of learning within creative development. The idea is that children are able to use a variety of ways to express themselves and that they gradually learn to talk about what they are doing.

Key messages in the Stepping Stones and Early Learning Goals

- **Senses** – this is the starting point with children being given opportunities to feel different textures and use different media. Eventually, children are expected to be able to talk about what they are feeling.
- **Use representation to communicate** – this comes in the blue Stepping Stone and is about children trying to express themselves and their ideas through media. This at first may mean making marks or building structures that have meaning for them.
- **Talk about their creations** – the idea is that children are able to talk about what they are doing and feeling, and explain their thoughts. A child may, for example, talk as they are painting or comment about how their model has turned out. Eventually, children will be able to evaluate their work and may be able to make suggestions as to how to improve or change what they have done.

Delivering this aspect of learning

This aspect of learning is about encouraging children to express themselves. The role of the adult is to support and provide opportunities. Adult-directed activities are clearly not appropriate here as the aim is for children to represent and express themselves in their chosen way. It will be important, however, for you to provide children with a range of textures, materials and ideas so that they can choose how best to put their ideas into shape.

Good practice checklist

◆ Are activities adult-directed or child-led?
◆ Are children encouraged to make their own choices about materials to use?
◆ Is a wide range of materials available for children to use?
◆ Do adults act as role models by using materials to create things for themselves?
◆ Do adults ask children about the process of creating rather than focusing on the end product?
◆ Are children given opportunities to look at each other's creations and to make comments about them?
◆ Is a range of sensory activities available, e.g. sand, water, malleable materials?

Specific activities for promoting creative development

Many of the Stepping Stones and Early Learning Goals for this area of learning can be delivered by adapting some basic activities.

Story bags

Story bags are one key way in which this area of learning can be promoted. Look for simple story lines that appeal to children. Read the book through several times so that children know the story by heart. Use props to animate the story and then make the bag available for children to use. Most children will wish to recreate the story using the same props. While commercially made bags are available, it is easy to devise your own. Hand-made bags have the advantage that you can tailor them to any story that you wish.

Musical games

Children can learn about what a range of percussion instruments can do by playing some simple games. They can, for example, play 'hot and cold' where one child is led to a hidden object by the others shaking their instruments loudly or being very quiet to show that the child has strayed from the object. It is also possible to combine story telling with instruments – for example, each child is given a character and plays their instrument as part of the story. Children also respond to musical games such as 'follow my leader' where they follow the rhythm of others.

Painting wall

Consider creating a large painting wall in your setting. This allows children to produce large paintings and also to paint alongside each other. Painting walls can be made by fixing plastic sheeting onto a wall with masking tape. Lining paper can then be taped onto the plastic sheeting so that children can paint or chalk on a large scale.

Dough, sand, water and paint

The traditional 'core activities' of early years settings are invaluable in delivering this area of learning. Children should be encouraged to enjoy the sensory experiences offered by these materials. They can also be shown how to 'tell' a story using these materials, e.g. 'Dinosaurs are lost in the sand – are they hiding or are they playing games?'

Valuing creative development

It is important that parents and adults in the setting understand that creative development is not always about taking things home. The process of creating must be valued for itself, as creativity is about expression rather than production.

Take photos or videos of children as they are 'creating' – use captions to explain how they are gaining in language development and social skills as well as learning to express themselves.

Send home notes or tell parents when their child has spent long periods of time being creative, e.g. playing with the story bag or playing in the home area.

Activity – Creative development

As part of this area of learning, children need to be given opportunities to make and use musical instruments.

Produce an activity plan for making simple musical instruments such as shakers. Your activity plan should explain:

◆ the resources required
◆ the role of the adult
◆ how this activity links to the Stepping Stones and Early Learning Goals.

Planning for the Foundation Stage

There are many systems of planning for the Foundation Stage. Whatever system you choose to adopt, it will be important to check that all the aspects of learning are being covered by the activities, routine and child-led play that your setting is offering.

◆ Read 'Planning for learning in the Foundation Stage' available free of charge from QCA ref. QCA/01/799.
◆ Find out if your local Early Years Childcare and Education Partnership has produced planning systems.
◆ Consider using some type of tracking to check that all aspects of learning are being provided for.
◆ In your planning consider putting the page numbers or a reference to the aspect of learning, Stepping Stone or Early Learning Goal that it is linked to.
◆ Remember that a theme-based approach to planning must be flexible enough to allow children to follow their own interests and also to avoid situations where valuable opportunities are lost because 'it doesn't fit with the theme'!
◆ Remember that activities that you are planning need to be play-based rather than formal learning.

Planning a balanced programme of activities

To achieve coverage of the curriculum and to promote individual children's interests and needs, it is a good idea to look at how your sessions are structured. Ideally, there should be several different types of activities going on alongside each other.

Area of learning	Activity	Key learning intentions + Key resources	Staff and children	Support required for individual children	Assessments of children's learning

An example of a session planner

Child-directed activities

These are activities that children choose and organise. They allow children to play at their own pace and build their confidence and skills. The adult may support and encourage but should not direct, so that children can explore in their own way.

Adult-structured activities

These are activities that the adult has structured to provide children with particular challenges and types of play. The adult may supervise and support, but does not necessarily take an active role.

Adult-directed activities

These activities are organised and led by adults so that children learn specific language or skills. For these types of activities to be successful, it is a good idea if adults work individually with children, or in very small groups, so that children can be actively involved.

A good approach is for the adult to direct an activity at first, but then encourage children to recreate the activity in their own way, e.g. an adult may show children how to blow bubbles, then leave them to practise and explore the mixture for themselves.

How can I order extra copies of the folder?

Copies of the folder ref. QCA/00/587 are available free of charge from QCA publications on 01787 884444. It is a good idea to consider ordering a folder for every member of staff, volunteers in your setting, and also some copies to lend out or to give to interested parents.

Part 2 Themes and activities for the Foundation Stage

Using themes

As part of developing children's learning, it has been a tradition among early years settings to plan play activities around a theme or a topic. This integrated approach to learning is useful as children's attention can be focused on a particular aspect of their world. Themes can help practitioners to channel their ideas and provide a focus in their planning. A theme is also a tool to involve parents, as they can see more clearly what they can build on at home, especially if you include a section in your planning that gives them suggestions on how to help their child at home.

This approach can still be used with the Foundation Stage curriculum, but the following points must be considered very carefully.

◆ How do the play activities link to and deliver the Foundation Stage curriculum?
◆ How will the play activities meet the needs of *all* children?
◆ Does the theme relate to children's experiences and everyday world?
◆ How will children's interests be followed?

These points highlight some of the difficulties of planning around a theme. In the past some settings have felt unable to carry out certain activities because they did not 'fit in with the theme'. A flexible approach must be taken so that we can be sure that all aspects of the Foundation Stage curriculum are being covered and, more importantly, that the activities offered to children meet their needs and interests.

Themes should reflect children's experiences

The themes that have been chosen in this section are not based on concepts, but are planned around children's experiences, particularly around objects that they can see and touch. This is likely to be a more useful approach than using concepts for themes. The danger with using a concept such as 'opposites' is that a child may not make the connections between the different planned activities. Themes that are planned directly around experiences and objects in children's lives are likely to have more relevance as they are 'concrete' and real for the child.

Seeing themes as 'starting points'

If you decide to deliver the Foundation Stage using themes or topics, it is important to see them only as starting points. Follow children's interests and see where they take you. You may, for example, start off with potatoes as your theme, but quickly find that children begin to talk about fruit, food or enjoy rolling the potatoes so much that you then plan activities that allow children to roll objects!

Some of a session's activities may centre around the theme, but others may not. Some activities that children enjoy doing and enhances their skills do not link to any particular theme. It is also likely that to deliver the Foundation Stage curriculum fully, you will need to provide some activities that do not link to themes.

Seeing the theme as a starting point also helps to make the theme more flexible – the best themes develop a life of their own as they follow the children's and the practitioner's interests. It also means that plans do not have to be a 'fixed' length and can be shortened or enlarged if necessary.

Choosing your own starting points

The best themes have meaning for children. They centre on things that young children are actually able to see, hold and touch. This means that children can use them in their play activities and learn *from* them, rather than just *about* them. A three year old, for example, will be able to hold a potato and do things with a potato, but will not be able to touch or hold 'growing' or 'opposite', which are concepts. Some traditional themes chosen by settings have been very 'adult' in nature and have been criticised because children have not made the associations between the activities, e.g. they have not understood that 'black and white' or 'up and down' are linked because they are opposites.

Run themes alongside other play activities

Children need a varied diet of play activities! Avoid thinking that only play activities that can be tied to a theme can be provided. Remember that all play is valid. If children want to play with dough and rolling pins, it does not matter whether it links to the theme or not. It is difficult and even unhealthy to try and link everything to a theme. If you take a flexible approach in your setting, you can gain the benefits of having a theme with the benefits of being child- and play-led.

Themes are unlikely to cover all aspects of learning

To deliver the Foundation Stage curriculum well, you will need to check that the various aspects of learning within each of the areas of learning are being covered regularly. ICT, for example, is an important aspect of learning that may not 'fit' with a theme, but nonetheless needs planning for. This is another reason for running themes in parallel with a range of other play activities.

How the themes in this book are organised

In this part of the book, a curriculum plan has been drawn up around a theme. Twenty activities have been put into the different areas of learning, although most will of course cover more than one area of learning. All the activities suggested on the curriculum plan should provide children with the opportunity to explore, be creative and to learn while having fun, enjoying the company of adults and other children, and playing.

For each theme six activities, one from each area of learning, have been discussed in more depth. These activities have been chosen because they can be adapted and used again with a different theme. They are divided into the following sections.

Specific resources

The key resources you will need in order to carry out the activity. Other resources such as aprons, protection for tables, may also be needed, but are likely to be put out automatically as part of the setting's routine.

Key learning intentions

Most activities will link to many areas of the Foundation Stage. The key learning intentions show the main focus of the activity.

Links to the Foundation Stage

This table shows the links to the Foundation Stage curriculum if the ideas for carrying out the activity are followed. The page reference will show you how the activity links to the Stepping Stones and Early Learning Goals and help you tailor the activity.

Ideas for organising the activity

This section provides suggestions as to how you may wish to organise an activity. It also suggests the group size. In many cases the activities work best with very small numbers of children at a time. This reflects the needs of young children who need time alone or in a small group with an adult in order to develop their language and to build up a relationship with other children. The Foundation Stage curriculum emphasises the need for children to talk freely about home and families and this is only likely to be achieved in situations where children are feeling relaxed and do not have to 'wait for their turn' to speak.

Extending and varying children's learning

Children's needs and interests vary considerably. This section gives some ideas of ways in which this activity could be extended, modified or reinforced.

Theme 1 Babies

Young children tend to know families with babies or have a baby in their own family. The starting point for this theme is the story *Avocado Baby* by John Burningham. As well as being funny, there are plenty of topics within the story. This is an excellent theme where a child has a newborn sibling.

   Inside the box on each area of learning below is a range of ideas for activities and stories on the theme of babies. You will find on the following pages a ready-made activity plan for the first idea listed in each box. In addition, all the stories mentioned are listed in the Booklist on pages 250–252.

Ideas to suggest to parents
- ◆ Show pictures of their child when s/he was a baby.
- ◆ Point out babies in prams and pushchairs when they are shopping.
- ◆ Visit a friend or neighbour who has a baby.

Personal, social and emotional development
- ◆ *Activity plan: Fruit tasting (p. 48)*
- ◆ Guess who was the baby? Display of photos of children and staff when they were babies.
- ◆ Teddy is feeling rather jealous of the new baby. Why is he feeling like this?
- ◆ Wash baby's clothes – why do we need to keep things clean?
- ◆ Stories:
  - ◆ *Avocado Baby*
  - ◆ *Owl Babies*

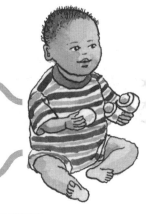

Communication, language and literacy
- ◆ *Activity plan: What can you do that babies can't? (p. 49)*
- ◆ Feely bag: What baby item can you feel?
- ◆ Role-play area: Baby cots, pushchairs, bottles, baby weighing clinic
- ◆ Songs rhymes and lullabies:
  - ◆ 'Pat-a-cake'
  - ◆ 'Peek-a-boo'
  - ◆ 'Rock-a bye baby'
- ◆ Stories:
  - ◆ *Avocado Baby*
  - ◆ *Baby Duck and the New Eyeglasses*
  - ◆ *Brand New Baby*
  - ◆ *Mr Davies and the Baby*
  - ◆ *Mrs Goose's Baby*
- ◆ Alliteration game: baby books, baby bites, baby baths – what others?
- ◆ Write a story about a baby going to sleep.
- ◆ Guess what this baby (doll) can do.
- ◆ Ask questions to see if you can find out about this baby's family.

Creative development

◆ *Activity plan: Don't wake the baby (p. 54)*
◆ Painting: pictures for the baby.
◆ Role play: Being a baby.
◆ Make up lullabies for babies: Can you make soothing sounds?
◆ Make a mobile to hang up in a room.
◆ Can you work out which rattle I am using to make this sound?
◆ Rattles, squeakers: what sounds can you make?

Physical development

◆ *Activity plan: Get baby home safely (p. 53)*
◆ Pram and pushchairs – keep them on the chalk lines.
◆ Sand tray, spoons and baby bowls – can you scoop and fill a baby's bowl?
◆ Baby beakers and bottles in the water tray: pouring.
◆ Teats, rings and bottles – can you screw the lids on the bottles?
◆ Can you dress the doll carefully and do up the poppers and buttons?
◆ How do babies show that they are tired? How do you show that you are tired?
◆ Fold baby's clothes.

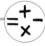

Knowledge and understanding of the world

◆ *Activity plan: Push and pull (p. 51)*
◆ How does your family celebrate the arrival of a baby? – photos of themselves and others as babies.
◆ Can you sort baby clothes that have poppers from ones that have buttons?
◆ Look at these baby toys – how do you make them work?
◆ Visit of a baby to the setting: What can the baby do? What does the baby need?

Mathematical development

◆ *Activity plan: Sorting baby clothes (p. 50)*
◆ Baby's bottles: Which bottle will empty the fastest? – use different flowing teats.
◆ Look at these baby dolls: Which is the heaviest? Which is the smallest?
◆ Scoops and sand: How many level scoops to fill the bottle?
◆ How many rattles in this feely bag – one, two, three or more?

Activity plans for the theme 'babies'

1 Fruit tasting

In the story *Avocado Baby*, the baby eats an avocado pear. This is a type of fruit. We have several different types of fruit for you to try. Which ones do you think you will like?

Specific resources

◆ avocado pear ◆ other fruit children may find interesting to taste
◆ ordinary pear ◆ sufficient plates and spoons to avoid possible cross-infection

Try approaching a supermarket for this activity as many will donate items.

Key learning intentions
This activity will help children to observe fruit carefully and talk about its taste, texture and appearance.

Links to Foundation Stage curriculum

Area of learning	Aspects of learning	Curriculum guidance page
Personal, social and emotional development	Disposition and attitudes Self-confidence and self-esteem Making relationships Behaviour and self-control Self-care	32 34 36 38 40
Communication, language and literacy	Language for communication Language for thinking Reading Writing Handwriting	48, 50, 52, 54 56–8 62 64 66
Mathematical development	Numbers as labels and for counting Calculating Shape, space and measures	74 76 78–80
Knowledge and understanding of the world	Exploration and investigation Cultures and beliefs	86, 88 98
Physical development	Health and bodily awareness Using equipment Using tools and materials	110 112 114
Creative development	Exploring media and materials Responding to experiences, and expressing and communicating ideas	120 126

Ideas for organising the activity

This activity works well with four children at a time, so that they can all talk and be active.

Show the different types of fruit to the children and ask them if they know the names of any of the fruits. Ask them to touch and gently hold the fruit. Model any new language for them, e.g. 'yes, yours is quite pale in colour'. Ask them if they can see any differences between the avocado pear and the 'real' pear. Write a label for each of the fruits so that the children see you write. With older children encourage them to say what the initial sound would be in the word.

Cut the fruit into halves and then into pieces. Can the children count the number of pieces? Put each type of fruit onto a separate plate and ask them if they can remember which label should go with which fruit.

The children can taste each type of fruit. Which one did they like the best? Why is fruit good for us? If the children are interested you might finish the activity by asking them to draw or 'write' down which fruit they enjoyed.

Health and safety
As with any food tasting activity, it is always important to check that children do not have any specific food allergies or dietary requirements.

Extending and varying children's learning
- Children write thank-you letters to the supermarket or shop that has donated the fruit.
- Plant the avocado stone.
- Produce some picture lotto cards with different types of fruit.
- Repeat the activity using dried fruits and fresh fruits, e.g. dried apple, fresh apple.

2 What can you do that babies can't?

Specific resources
- paper and crayons
- photos of children and babies (could be of the children themselves)

Key learning intentions
This activity helps children to use language to talk about differences and about things that have happened in the past. It will also develop early reading and writing skills.

Links to Foundation Stage curriculum

Area of learning	Aspects of learning	Curriculum guidance page
Personal, social and emotional development	Disposition and attitudes Self-confidence and self-esteem Making relationships Self-care Sense of community	32 34 36 40 42

Communication, language and literacy	Language for communication	48, 50, 52, 54
	Language for thinking	56–8
	Linking sounds with letters	60
	Reading	62
	Writing	64
Knowledge and understanding of the world	Designing and making skills	90
	Sense of time	94
Physical development	Using equipment	112
	Using tools and materials	114
Creative development	Responding to experiences, and expressing and communicating ideas	126

Ideas for organising the activity

This activity will work well with small groups of children, pairs, as well as with individual children. Read the story *Avocado Baby*. Ask the children: 'What can the baby in the story do? Is this what most babies do? What do babies do? What can children do now that they could not do when they were babies?' Use the photos of babies and children to help prompt children's ideas, e.g. a photo of a child drawing – can babies draw?

   Ask children to draw pictures of the things that they can do, but babies cannot do. Encourage them to 'write' about their pictures. Use the photos, pictures and mark making children have produced to build up a display. Encourage them to write their names on their work or to find their name cards.

Extending and varying children's learning

◆ Children can make a collage of baby pictures.
◆ Encourage children to act out looking after a baby, especially if a baby has visited the setting.

3 Sorting baby clothes

Look at these baby clothes. They are all different sizes. Can we work out which ones are for a newborn baby?

Specific resources

◆ a range of baby clothes, preferably: newborn, 6–12 months and 18 months (aim to provide clothes that reflect different family traditions)

> **Key learning intentions**
> This activity helps children to sort, match and count. They will also be using fine motor skills to fold and sort clothes.

Links to Foundation Stage curriculum		
Area of learning	**Aspects of learning**	**Curriculum guidance page**
Personal, social and emotional development	Disposition and attitudes Self-confidence and self-esteem Making relationships Behaviour and self-control Self-care Sense of community	32 34 36 38 40 42
Communication, language and literacy	Language for communication Language for thinking	48, 50, 52, 54 56–8
Mathematical development	Numbers as labels and for counting Calculating Shape, space and measures	74 76 78–80
Knowledge and understanding of the world	Exploration and investigation Sense of time Cultures and beliefs	86, 88 94 98
Physical development	Movement Health and bodily awareness Using tools and materials	106, 108 110 114

Ideas for organising the activity

This activity can be done with pairs of children at a time, or even small groups. Show children the different types of baby clothes. Ask them to tell you what each item is called and what it is used for, e.g. a bonnet is used to keep the head warm. Bring into the discussion the importance of dressing for the weather, e.g. sunhats in the summer.

Encourage children to choose their favourite items. Why do they like them – is it the colour, the feel or the design? Ask them if they could sort out the clothes into three piles – small, medium and large. Encourage them to do this together. How many is there in each pile?

Extending and varying children's learning

- Encourage further sorting by putting the clothes out as part of the role-play area.
- Children can 'write' a note to say which pile has the smallest clothes in it.
- Produce a display showing small, medium and large.
- Encourage children to put the clothes against themselves.
- See if children can work out the order in which a baby would be dressed.

4 Push and pull

The avocado baby was so strong that it could push the family's car. Can you make your own car that could be pushed?

Specific resources

- boxes
- lids
- paper
- crayons
- staplers
- sticky tape
- clingfilm
- other materials for junk modelling

Key learning intentions
The aim of this activity is to encourage children's designing and making skills as well as their creativity.

Links to Foundation Stage curriculum

Area of learning	Aspects of learning	Curriculum guidance page
Personal, social and emotional development	Disposition and attitudes Making relationships Behaviour and self-control Self-care	32 36 38 40
Communication, language and literacy	Language for communication Language for thinking Writing	48, 50, 52, 54 56–8 64
Mathematical development	Calculating Shape, space and measures	76 78–80
Knowledge and understanding of the world	Exploration and investigation Designing and making skills	86, 88 90
Physical development	Using equipment Using tools and materials	112 114
Creative development	Exploring media and materials Imagination Responding to experiences, and expressing and communicating ideas	120 124 126

Ideas for organising the activity

This activity works best with two or three children at a time, as adult support will be required to help children design and then make their own car.

Start by showing children different ways of making a box move, e.g. lids with a stick pushed through the centre, using wheels from a set. Show them the range of materials available and see if they have any ideas how they could be transformed, e.g. this could be a window. Avoid imposing your own ideas of how a car should look! For this to be a creative activity, the role of the adult must be supportive not directive. Children will need plenty of time as some will want to play with the materials as they work.

When they have finished ask them if they would like to 'make their mark' on a sticky label so that you will know that it is theirs. Provide name cards if necessary to help children remember the shape of the letters in their names.

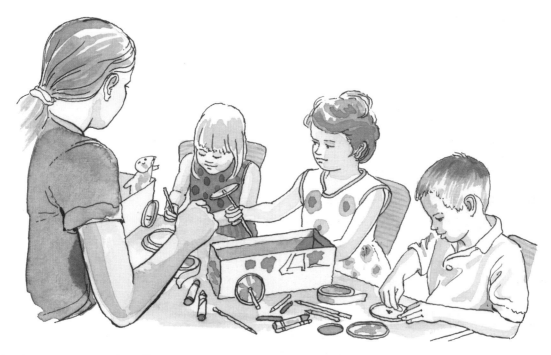

Avoid imposing your own ideas of how a car should look!

If possible provide the children with 'play people' so that they can re-enact the story of the baby pushing the family in the car.

Extending and varying children's learning

◆ Encourage the children to play with their cars.
◆ See which cars roll or can be pushed.
◆ Ask the children to make other cars using construction equipment such as Duplo and Lego.
◆ See which car will roll the furthest.
◆ Look at toy cars – sort out the cars which are green like the one in the book.

5 Get baby home safely

Let's make an obstacle course and then see if you can take your baby doll or teddy safely around it.

Specific resources

◆ equipment such as hoops, play tunnels, cushions, mats, benches

---

Key learning intentions
This activity is designed to develop children's gross motor and locomotive skills. It should also help develop their spatial awareness.

Links to Foundation Stage curriculum		
Area of learning	**Aspects of learning**	**Curriculum guidance page**
Personal, social and emotional development	Disposition and attitudes Self-confidence and self-esteem Making relationships Behaviour and self-control Self-care	32 34 36 38 40
Communication, language and literacy	Language for communication	48, 50, 52, 54
Mathematical development	Shape, space and measures	78–80
Knowledge and understanding of the world	Exploration and investigation Designing and making skills	86, 88 90
Physical development	Sense of space Movement Health and bodily awareness Using equipment	104 106, 108 110 112
Creative development	Exploring media and materials Imagination	120 124

Ideas for organising the activity

Begin by setting up a simple obstacle course either in or out of doors. Can the children pick up a doll or teddy and take it around with them?

Ask small groups or pairs of children if they would like to add to or change the obstacle course. Encourage the use of positional language such as 'alongside', 'under' or 'on top of'. Many children will also want to 'role play', taking the baby or cuddly toy along the trail.

Extending and varying children's learning

- Children can take it in turns to go on each other's obstacle course.
- Children can then 'draw' the trail.
- Use this activity as a starting point for 'walks', e.g. read the book *Rosie's Walk*.
- Hide or put objects to do with babies along the obstacle course for children to pick up.

6 Don't wake the baby

Let's imagine that there is a baby fast asleep. We have to creep around trying to be quiet, but sometimes we suddenly make lots of noise! Then one of us has to rock the baby and get it back to sleep.

Specific resources
◆ *Don't Wake the Baby* by Francesca Simon
◆ a range of percussion instruments
◆ a doll in a cot

Key learning intentions
This activity is designed to help children learn to ask questions and to expand their vocabulary. They will also be learning to co-operate with others and to listen carefully.

Links to Foundation Stage curriculum		
Area of learning	**Aspects of learning**	**Curriculum guidance page**
Personal, social and emotional development	Disposition and attitudes Making relationships	32 36
Communication, language and literacy	Language for communication Language for thinking	48, 50, 52, 54 56–8
Mathematical development	Numbers as labels and for counting Shape, space and measures	74 78–80
Knowledge and understanding of the world	Exploration and investigation Information and communication technology Sense of time	86, 88 92 94
Physical development	Movement Using tools and materials	106, 108 114
Creative development	Exploring media and materials Music Imagination	120 122 124

Ideas for organising the activity
This activity will work well with small groups of children. Begin by reading them the story of how everyone in the family was trying to keep quiet. Ask the children if they would like to play a game. Bring out the musical instruments for the children to explore. Encourage them to see what sounds they make. Place the doll on your lap. Tell the children that they can move around with the instruments, but when you put the baby in the cot, they should try and move as quietly as possible. Keep picking up the baby and putting down the baby as part of the game.

Extending and varying children's learning
◆ Encourage children to take it in turns to play the part of the parent putting the baby to sleep.
◆ Sing lullabies and encourage the children to use the instruments to make soothing sounds.
◆ Ask children to choose the instrument that they think the baby would like the most.

Theme 2 Bags

'Bags' is a good theme because nearly all children will have used a bag or seen a bag being used. As a starting point, it could be used to look at journeys or shops.

Inside the box on each area of learning below is a range of ideas for activities and stories on the theme of bags. You will find on the following pages a ready-made activity plan for the first idea listed in each box. In addition, all the stories mentioned are listed in the Booklist on pages 250–252.

Ideas to suggest to parents
- ◆ Encourage their child to look at the different types of bag they use in the house.
- ◆ See if their child can recognise any of the 'brand' names on carrier bags.
- ◆ Encourage their child to pack their own bag to come into the setting.

Personal, social and emotional development
- ◆ *Activity plan: I went to the shops and I bought … (p. 58)*
- ◆ Bags you have at home.
- ◆ Bags that you can and cannot play with.
- ◆ Tidy out the toy cupboard – put unwanted or things to be mended in the bags.

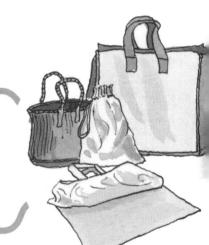

Communication, language and literacy
- ◆ *Activity plan: What's the story? (p. 59)*
- ◆ Guess what is in the feely bag.
- ◆ Story bags: Can you work out which story this bag is for?
- ◆ Role-play area: Supermarkets.
- ◆ Which bag does this belong in?
- ◆ Make a shopping list.
- ◆ I am thinking of a bag – can you guess which one of these it is?

Creative development

- *Activity plan: Make a lucky dip bag (p. 64)*
- Listen to the sound that I am making in the bag – what do you think made it?
- Let's pretend to go shopping – when the music stops, find something to put in your bag.
- Put your hands in this bag – can you draw how it feels to you? Is it soft, sticky or cold?
- Role-play area: Suitcase and bag shop.

Physical development

- *Activity plan: Pack a bag for teddy (p. 63)*
- Playing with sacks/sleeping bags – can you wiggle like a worm?
- Can you deliver this shopping? – You can use tricycles, prams or walk with it.
- Put a balloon inside a cloth bag – how far can you throw it?
- Parachute game – run into the middle when you hear your 'bag' name.
- Fold up this sheet – which bag can you get it in?
- Can you throw any beanbags into that large bag?

Knowledge and understanding of the world

- *Activity plan: Which is the strongest bag for teddy's shopping? (p. 61)*
- Do you recognise these bags – where are they from?
- Sort bags – which have handles, which have straps?
- Sort bags according to materials.
- Make a bag for teddy to keep his pens and pencils in.
- Bring in some of the bags you use at home – when do you use them?
- Let's put some water into this bag – let's see what happens when it freezes.

Mathematical development
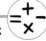

- *Activity plan: The bags game (p. 60)*
- Can you order these bags according to size?
- Which of these bags will hold the most?
- Shop: Can you count the coins into the bags?
- Can you find things that are heavier than this bag of flour?
- How many bags inside this bag?
- Find the bag with one item, two items, three items … five items.
- Which of these bags is the heaviest? Which is the lightest?

Activity plans for the theme 'bags'

1 I went to the shops and I bought ...

Let's play a shopping game. In this game you have to remember what everyone has bought.

Specific resources

◆ a range of objects that can be bought in a shop, e.g. bananas, cuddly toys, games, clothes

---

Key learning intentions

This activity is designed to help children co-operate together while also helping them use recall and sequencing.

Links to Foundation Stage curriculum		
Area of learning	**Aspects of learning**	**Curriculum guidance page**
Personal, social and emotional development	Disposition and attitudes Self-confidence and self-esteem Making relationships Behaviour and self-control Sense of community	32 34 36 38 42
Communication, language and literacy	Language for communication Language for thinking	48, 50, 52, 54 56–8
Mathematical development	Numbers as labels and for counting	74
Knowledge and understanding of the world	Sense of time	94
Creative development	Imagination	124

Ideas for organising the activity

This activity works well with a group size of around six to eight children. Begin by arranging the children in a circle with the objects that you have chosen in the middle. Take an object, e.g. a banana, and say 'I went to the shop and I bought a banana.'

Ask the child next to you to take another object. Encourage all the children to say together 'I went to the shop and I bought a banana and a (next object).' The game continues with each child taking an item and the chant getting longer. They will be helped to remember what was taken by seeing the objects in the hands of the other children.

Extending and varying children's learning

◆ Children can play this game, but remember for themselves the order of objects.
◆ Put out unusual objects so that children's vocabulary is extended.
◆ Produce a shopping list with pictures so that children take an object according to the list.

2 What's the story?

Look in this bag. What items are inside? Can we make a story up?

Specific resources
◆ fabric bag
◆ cuddly toy
◆ three or four small items children will be familiar with

Key learning intentions
This activity will help develop children's language, especially vocabulary, and their ability to use talk to organise their thinking.

Links to Foundation Stage curriculum

Area of learning	Aspects of learning	Curriculum guidance page
Personal, social and emotional development	Disposition and attitudes Self-confidence and self-esteem Making relationships	32 34 36
Communication, language and literacy	Language for communication Language for thinking	48, 50, 52, 54 56–8
Mathematical development	Numbers as labels and for counting	74
Knowledge and understanding of the world	Exploration and investigation	86, 88
Physical development	Using tools and materials	114
Creative development	Imagination Responding to experiences, and expressing and communicating ideas	124 126

Ideas for organising the activity

This activity works well with pairs or small groups of children so they can put forward their ideas easily.

Begin by showing children the objects in the bag. Can they take them out and name them? Allow them to touch, explore and talk about what is there. Choose objects that are interesting, but are recognisable by children. To make it easier, items can be connected in some way, e.g. items associated with the seaside or with gardening.

Introduce the cuddly toy to the children – he has been using these items. Encourage them to talk about what they think he has been doing. Encourage children to touch the items as they are speaking about them.

Extending and varying children's learning
◆ Encourage children to draw pictures or to 'write the story'.
◆ Vary this activity by encouraging children to choose items for the bag for you to tell a story with.
◆ Bring in unusual items and explain their purpose to children.

3 The bags game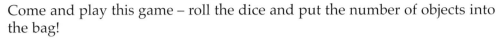

Come and play this game – roll the dice and put the number of objects into the bag!

Specific resources

◆ bags – paper, fabric or plastic (providing game is supervised and bags have holes in them)
◆ dice
◆ small objects, e.g. counters, buttons, shells, toy cars, etc.

Key learning intentions
This activity will help number recognition and use of numbers for counting.

Links to Foundation Stage curriculum

Area of learning	Aspects of learning	Curriculum guidance page
Personal, social and emotional development	Disposition and attitudes	32
Communication, language and literacy	Language for communication Language for thinking	48, 50, 52, 54 56–8
Mathematical development	Numbers as labels and for counting Calculating Shape, space and measures	74 76 78–80
Knowledge and understanding of the world	Exploration and investigation	86, 88
Physical development	Using tools and materials	114

Ideas for organising the activity

This activity works well with pairs or small groups of children. Begin by letting them play with the objects you have chosen. Will they all fit in the bags? Can they recognise the numbers shown on the bags? (If at this point children do not recognise the numerals, consider changing the activity. The dice can be adapted so that instead of numbers it shows colours – children have coloured bags and choose the right coloured object to go into the bag.)

Each child has six numbered bags. They roll the dice and then count objects out to that number. They then put the objects into the correct bag. Once all of their bags have been filled they have won the game.

Extending and varying children's learning

◆ Encourage children to play the game in pairs.
◆ Change the game so that children begin with a number of objects in a single bag and then take them away according to the number shown on the dice.
◆ Encourage children to choose their own objects for the game.

4 Which is the strongest bag for teddy's shopping?

Look at these three bags – which do you think will be the strongest?

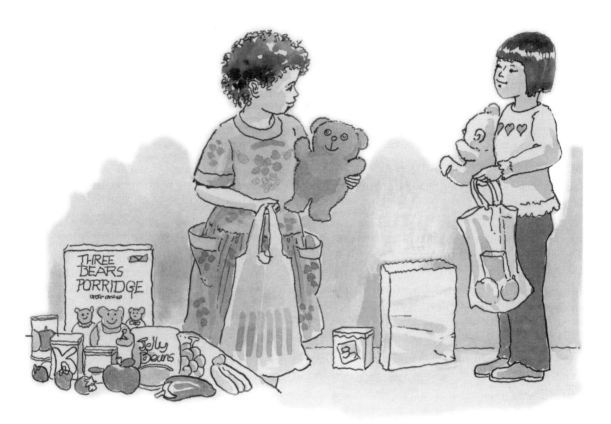

Which will be the easiest one to carry home?

Specific resources

◆ thin carrier bag
◆ paper bag
◆ strong carrier bag

◆ items of shopping, e.g. tins, boxes, fruit
◆ teddy bear or cuddly toy

> **Key learning intentions**
> This activity is designed to encourage children to look at the properties of materials and to consider ways of testing materials.

Links to Foundation Stage curriculum		
Area of learning	**Aspects of learning**	**Curriculum guidance page**
Personal, social and emotional development	Disposition and attitudes	32
Communication, language and literacy	Language for communication Language for thinking	48, 50, 52, 54 56–8
Mathematical development	Shape, space and measures	78–80
Knowledge and understanding of the world	Exploration and investigation Designing and making skills	86, 88 90
Physical development	Movement Using tools and materials	106, 108 114
Creative development	Exploring media and materials	120

Ideas for organising the activity

This activity works well with pairs of children or small groups. Begin by showing them the three different bags. Do they know where they came from or what they might be used for?

Tell the children that teddy needs to choose one bag to take his shopping home in. Encourage them to talk about the items that teddy has bought – do they buy any of these when they go shopping? Ask the children to decide which bag the shopping should go in – does the bag feel strong enough? Try out all three bags – how do they compare? Which will be the easiest one to carry home?

Health and safety

Use this as a reinforcement activity that children should never put plastic bags over their heads. To avoid any danger to children, use carrier bags that have been perforated.

Extending and varying children's learning

- Children can write to teddy's mum telling her that he has bought the shopping.
- Children can repeat this activity in the role-play area, but using different bags, e.g. baskets, larger paper bags.
- Children can repeat this activity looking at which bags will hold the most.
- Ask children to think about how best to pack a bag so that soft items do not get squashed.
- Children can take teddy around the role-play 'supermarket' with a shopping list and help him find his shopping.

5 Pack a bag for teddy 🏋

Teddy is going away to his friend's. He needs to pack his bag of clothes. Can you help him?

Specific resources
- holdall or sports bag
- clothes
- toiletries

Key learning intentions

This activity should help children's fine motor skills as they fold clothes carefully.

Links to Foundation Stage curriculum		
Area of learning	**Aspects of learning**	**Curriculum guidance page**
Personal, social and emotional development	Disposition and attitudes Self-confidence and self-esteem Making relationships Behaviour and self-control Self-care	32 34 36 38 40
Communication, language and literacy	Language for communication Language for thinking Handwriting	48, 50, 52, 54 56–8 66
Mathematical development	Numbers as labels and for counting Shape, space and measures	74 78–80
Knowledge and understanding of the world	Exploration and investigation	86, 88
Physical development	Movement Using tools and materials	106 114
Creative development	Exploring media and materials Imagination Responding to experiences, and expressing and communicating ideas	120 124 126

Ideas for organising the activity

This activity works best with individual children or pairs.

Begin by showing children teddy and the holdall. Ask them if they would like to pack his holdall by folding his clothes. Encourage them to count and talk about the uses of the clothes that teddy needs packing. You may need to show them how to fold some clothes – this can be done in a fun way by pretending that you are explaining and showing teddy.

Use this activity as a way of encouraging children to talk about any trips or holidays that they have taken. They may also talk about clothes that they enjoy wearing at home.

Extending and varying children's learning

◆ Ask the children to write a note to teddy's mum explaining that the packing has been done.
◆ Encourage children to pack some toys for teddy to play with.
◆ Encourage children to choose other clothes and items for teddy.

6 Make a lucky dip bag

Look at these lovely bits and pieces. Would you like to choose some to put into a lucky dip bag?

Specific resources

◆ paper
◆ crayons
◆ small items for surprises
◆ sticky tape

Key learning intentions
This activity will help children to design and construct whilst exploring properties of materials.

Links to Foundation Stage curriculum		
Area of learning	**Aspects of learning**	**Curriculum guidance page**
Personal, social and emotional development	Disposition and attitudes Self-confidence and self-esteem Making relationships Behaviour and self-control Self-care Sense of community	32 34 36 38 40 42
Communication, language and literacy	Language for communication Language for thinking Writing	48, 50, 52, 54 56–8 64
Mathematical development	Numbers as labels and for counting Shape, space and measures	74 78–80
Knowledge and understanding of the world	Exploration and investigation Designing and making skills	86, 88 90
Physical development	Movement Using tools and materials	106, 108 114
Creative development	Exploring media and materials Imagination Responding to experiences, and expressing and communicating ideas	120 124 126

Ideas for organising the activity

This activity works well with pairs or individual children. Begin by asking children if they know what a lucky dip bag is. Ask them if they like surprises. Then ask them to choose an item and make a bag for it. Encourage them to think of their own ways of making a bag. This may mean supporting them, giving a little guidance. Avoid giving them too many directions.

Encourage children to choose ways of decorating their bags. The bags can then be put together for all the children in the setting to take one at random or, if they want their own bag, they can take it home!

Extending and varying children's learning

◆ Encourage children to prepare lucky dip bags that can be sold to raise money for a charity or for the setting.

◆ Provide other objects for children to 'wrap' up in a bag.

◆ Play games where children have to guess what is in a bag by feeling it.

Theme 3 Books

A love of books is essential if children are to become keen readers. This theme acts as a good starting point to help children and their parents focus on books. Encourage children to bring in books they enjoy at home and try and get a range of different types of books for them to explore.

Inside the box on each area of learning below is a range of ideas for activities and stories on the theme of books. You will find on the following pages a ready-made activity plan for the first idea listed in each box. In addition, all the stories mentioned are listed in the Booklist on pages 250–252.

Ideas to suggest to parents

◆ Take their child to the library.

◆ Talk about different types of books that they have.

◆ Borrow one of our books to share with their child.

◆ Show their child any books that are special in their family, e.g. baby album.

Personal, social and emotional development

◆ *Activity plan: Repairing books (p. 68)*

◆ Books that make me feel good.

◆ Bring in a favourite book from home.

◆ Share a book with a friend.

◆ Make a display of your favourite books.

◆ Cleaning and tidying the story area.

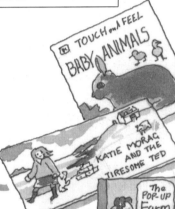

Communication, language and literacy

◆ *Activity plan: Can you match the pictures with the book? (p. 69)*

◆ Choose a book to share with an adult.

◆ Sequencing – can you work out the order of this story?

◆ Role-play area: At the bookshop.

◆ Let's make up our own story: Look at these objects – where do they come from?

◆ Books that begin with 'Once upon a time'.

◆ Stories:
  ◆ *Each Peach Pear Plum*
  ◆ *Finish the Story, Dad*
  ◆ *I Like Books*
  ◆ *Just One More Story*

◆ Look at books: Which ones have animals in them?

◆ I am thinking of a book … can you find it?

◆ Use a recipe book – can we follow these instructions?

Creative development

- ◆ *Activity plan: Make a flap book (p. 73)*
- ◆ Make a bookmark.
- ◆ Draw pictures of our favourite books and characters.
- ◆ Role-play area: At the library.
- ◆ Make a library for the small world people.

Physical development

- ◆ *Activity plan: Books that I like at bedtime (p. 72)*
- ◆ Can you fold these sheets of paper to make a book?
- ◆ Look at these pop-up books – can you handle them carefully?
- ◆ Tidy books on the bookshelf.
- ◆ Parachute game: You are a type of book – when your type is called, run around the outside of the parachute.

Knowledge and understanding of the world

- ◆ *Activity plan: Let's make a book about this setting (p. 71)*
- ◆ Make our own library cards.
- ◆ Let's make a book about your day.
- ◆ Where can we find books in this area?
- ◆ Visit a library.
- ◆ Ask a librarian in to talk to us.
- ◆ Sort books out according to type.
- ◆ Special books in our families.
- ◆ Make our own recipe book – can you bring in a favourite recipe from home?

Mathematical development

- ◆ *Activity plan: The bookshop game (p. 70)*
- ◆ Can you order these books according to height?
- ◆ Which of these books is the smallest?
- ◆ Which of these three books is the heaviest? Which is the lightest?
- ◆ Which of these books have page numbers?
- ◆ Make a book that is small enough to go in teddy's tiny box.

Activity plans for the theme 'books'

I Repairing books

I am going to repair these books, would you like to help as well?

Specific resources

- damaged books
- books to be covered with plastic
- sticky backed plastic
- sticky tape
- scissors

Key learning intentions

This activity helps children learn about taking care of their immediate environment, and to develop the skill of using scissors. It is a chance to build a relationship with an adult.

Links to Foundation Stage curriculum

Area of learning	Aspects of learning	Curriculum guidance page
Personal, social and emotional development	Disposition and attitudes Behaviour and self-control	32 38
Communication, language and literacy	Language for communication Language for thinking	48, 50, 52, 54 56–8
Mathematical development	Numbers as labels and for counting Calculating Shape, space and measures	74 76 78–80
Physical development	Sense of space Movement Using equipment	104 106, 108 112

Ideas for organising the activity

This activity works best with individual children or pairs.

Begin by showing children what needs doing, looking at books and working out how to repair them. Use this as an opportunity to talk about why books might become damaged and how to avoid damage. Show children how you repair books, measuring sticky tape, and encourage them to try this out.

The focus of this activity is to find ways of listening to children and while you may begin by talking about books and things that get broken, they may also want to use this as an opportunity to talk about themselves and things that are important to them.

Extending and varying children's learning

- Have a book sale – children can bring in books, repair them and then sell them.
- Show other children in the group the books that have been repaired.
- Involve children in other 'adult' activities such as washing up or tidying away.

2 Can you match the pictures with the book?

Look at these pictures – do you recognise the book they are from?

Specific resources

◆ pictures (cut off the text) from damaged books that have been popular with children (these can be laminated for durability)
◆ 'whole' books so that children can be read the whole story

Key learning intentions
This activity will encourage children to draw and 'write' as well as to 'retell' the story.

Links to Foundation Stage curriculum

Area of learning	Aspects of learning	Curriculum guidance page
Personal, social and emotional development	Disposition and attitudes	32
Communication, language and literacy	Language for communication Language for thinking	48, 50, 52, 54 56–8
Mathematical development	Shape, space and measures	78–80
Knowledge and understanding of the world	Designing and making skills Information and communication technology	90 92
Physical development	Using tools and materials	114
Creative development	Exploring media and materials Responding to experiences, and expressing and communicating ideas	120 126

Ideas for organising the activity

This activity works well with pairs or individual children. Begin by reading the 'whole' book to children. Encourage them to talk about the book.

Show the children the laminated pictures. Can they match these pictures to the pages in the 'whole' book? Can they tell you what is happening in these pictures?

Ask the children if they can 'write' on a piece of paper the words in their own writing. Encourage children to feel confident by praising their attempts at mark making.

Extending and varying children's learning

◆ Can they draw some more pictures about the story?
◆ If you have several pictures from one story can they put them in the correct order?
◆ Can they tell the story to 'teddy' or another child?

3 The bookshop game

Let's play the bookshop game. Here are some books. Roll the dice – how many books are sold?

Specific resources
◆ books
◆ dice or cards showing the number of books to be taken

Key learning intentions
This activity is designed to help children use numbers as labels and to use subtraction in a practical way.

Links to Foundation Stage curriculum		
Area of learning	**Aspects of learning**	**Curriculum guidance page**
Personal, social and emotional development	Disposition and attitudes	32
Communication, language and literacy	Language for communication Language for thinking Writing	48, 50, 52, 54 56–8 64
Creative development	Imagination Responding to experiences, and expressing and communicating ideas	124 126

Ideas for organising the activity
This activity works best with groups of three or four children. Change the dice, using stickers so that only numbers 1–3 are shown. Ask the children to choose about ten books each – you may need to count them with the children. Which ones are their favourites?

Ask them if they can put the books into a pile in front of them. Tell them that they have now set up their own bookshop! Explain that when the dice is rolled they will put the number of books shown by the dice into the middle as these books have now been sold. The first person to sell all their books is the winner.

This game can be made simpler by putting drawings of books onto cards. The children can then take the number of books away that is shown on the cards.

Extending and varying children's learning
◆ Play a game where children put a coin in the middle each time a book is sold.
◆ Vary the game by playing libraries – some books are taken away, others are brought back.
◆ Ask children to count how many books there are – can they put the books into pairs?
◆ Encourage children to sort books – which ones have page numbers on them?

4 Let's make a book about this setting

We do lots of lovely things here. Wouldn't it be nice to make a book about us?

Specific resources

- camera
- pens
- glue
- photographs
- paper
- staplers
- pencils
- scissors
- puppet or teddy

Key learning intentions

This activity helps children think more about their immediate environment as well as helping them to see that they are part of a community.

Links to Foundation Stage curriculum		
Area of learning	**Aspects of learning**	**Curriculum guidance page**
Personal, social and emotional development	Disposition and attitudes Self-confidence and self-esteem Making relationships Behaviour and self-control Sense of community	32 34 36 38 42
Communication, language and literacy	Language for communication Language for thinking	48, 50, 52, 54 56–8
Knowledge and understanding of the world	Sense of time Sense of place	94 96
Physical development	Sense of space Movement	104 106, 108

Ideas for organising the activity

This activity works well with two or three children at a time, though the finished book should be contributed to by each child.

Start the activity using a new stooge such as a puppet or teddy. Tell the children that s/he does not know anything about the setting – could we make a book for him/her about the setting? Encourage them to talk to the puppet or teddy about what they enjoy doing in the setting as well as about each other and the outside of the building.

Ask them what they would like to do to help make a book, e.g. take photographs, choose pictures, draw pictures, etc. (Note that by taking photographs children will be practising their ICT skills.) Once all the children have made a contribution, share the book with small groups. Can they see their photograph or the page that they helped with? Display the book for parents to see and encourage children to look at it.

Extending and varying children's learning

- Children take photographs for their own book.
- Play a game where children have to find a certain page in the book, e.g. the outside of the book.
- Children talk about the book to the stooge.

5 Books that I like at bedtime

What book do you like to share at bedtime? Shall we look at some of our favourites?

Specific resources
- books children have brought in
- books about bedtime
- cuddly toys
- teddy bears
- blankets
- toy cots or beds

Key learning intentions
This activity is designed to help children to recognise being tired and talk about ways of resting.

Links to Foundation Stage curriculum

Area of learning	Aspects of learning	Curriculum guidance page
Personal, social and emotional development	Disposition and attitudes Self-confidence and self-esteem Sense of community	32 34 42
Communication, language and literacy	Language for communication Language for thinking	48, 50, 52, 54 56–8
Mathematical development	Numbers as labels and for counting Calculating Shape, space and measures	74 76 78–80
Physical development	Using equipment Using tools and materials	112 114
Creative development	Imagination	124

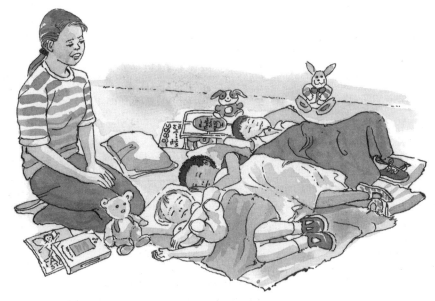

Encourage them to talk about feeling tired and how they get to sleep

Ideas for organising the activity

This activity works well with pairs or small groups. Ask children if they have brought in their favourite bedtime reading. Encourage them to talk about feeling tired and how they get to sleep. Read stories about bedtimes, e.g. *Can't You Sleep, Little Bear?*

Talk to children about what happens if the body does not get enough sleep. Use this activity as a way of helping children talk about their homes and their routines.

Extending and varying children's learning

◆ Ask children to think about other things that help them to rest and sleep.
◆ Use a puppet or teddy and talk about what happens when you are feeling tired.
◆ Put books about bedtime into the role-play area so that children can put dolls, teddies and other cuddly toys to sleep.

6 Make a flap book

Did you enjoy the flap book? Would you like to make your own flap book?

Specific resources

◆ flap book
◆ glue
◆ paper
◆ pens
◆ sticky tape
◆ pencils and crayons

> *Key learning intentions*
> This activity is designed to help children learn how to make a flap book.

Links to Foundation Stage curriculum		
Area of learning	**Aspects of learning**	**Curriculum guidance page**
Personal, social and emotional development	Disposition and attitudes Self-confidence and self-esteem Making relationships Behaviour and self-control	32 34 36 38
Communication, language and literacy	Language for communication Language for thinking Reading Writing Handwriting	48, 50, 52, 54 56–8 62 64 66
Mathematical development	Shape, space and measures	78–80
Knowledge and understanding of the world	Designing and making skills	90
Physical development	Using tools and materials	114
Creative development	Exploring media and materials Imagination Responding to experiences, and expressing and communicating ideas	120 124 126

Ideas for organising the activity

This activity can be carried out with individual children or very small groups. Begin by putting out a collection of simple flap books that children might enjoy, e.g. *Where's Spot?* Show children how, by putting a piece of paper over a picture and attaching the top edge either with sticky tape or glue, it will make a flap. Ask the children if they would like to make their own flap books or pictures. Encourage children to choose materials that they would like to use to make the book and what type of things might be hidden under a flap. The key to this activity is to encourage children to talk about their own 'story' and also to allow children to work out for themselves how best to make the 'flaps'. The role of the adult is to support children; for example, by holding the sticky tape so that children can cut it, rather than to make the book for the child.

Extending and varying children's learning

- ◆ Encourage children to 'write' their story down in their own way.
- ◆ Display the children's work in the book area.
- ◆ Encourage children to 'read' or 'tell' their story.
- ◆ Ask children to find their favourite 'flap' book.

Theme 4 Boxes

Most young children have seen and handled boxes. It is a theme that has many starting points as some children are fascinated by boxes. Consider using this as a theme if a child is moving house, it's near Christmas or a festival where presents are exchanged.

Inside the box on each area of learning below is a range of ideas for activities and stories on the theme of boxes. You will find on the following pages a ready-made activity plan for the first idea listed in each box. In addition, all the stories mentioned are listed in the Booklist on pages 250–252.

Ideas to suggest to parents
- ◆ Let their child play with a box big enough for them to sit inside.
- ◆ Point out boxes and packaging when they are shopping.
- ◆ Help their child to make a box for their toys.

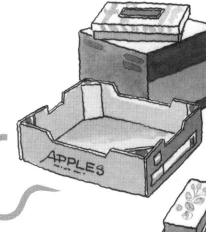

Personal, social and emotional development

- ◆ *Activity plan: A shoebox of memories (p. 78)*
- ◆ Caring for our environment – tidying and sorting out things into boxes.
- ◆ Looking after special things – special boxes.
- ◆ Are there any boxes and bottles that we must not touch?
- ◆ Can you put these toys back into the right boxes?

Communication, language and literacy

- ◆ *Activity plan: Guess what's in my box! (p. 79)*
- ◆ Role-play area: Box shop – guess what is in the boxes?
- ◆ Kim's game: Which box has disappeared?
- ◆ Put the objects beginning with the letter 'b' inside the box.
- ◆ Box treasure hunt – which of these boxes has your name written inside?
- ◆ What has teddy got in his special box?
- ◆ Story: *Maisy Dresses Up*

Creative development

◆ *Activity plan: Make a puppet theatre from a box (p. 84)*

◆ Can you make/decorate your own special box for your treasures?

◆ Can you make a Jack-in-the-box?

◆ Small boxes to use as shakers.

◆ Musical boxes – dance when you can hear the music.

◆ Show me all the things that you can do with this box in the sand tray.

Physical development

◆ *Activity plan: Sandcastle boxes (p. 83)*

◆ Tiny boxes in sandpit: scooping, hiding objects, hiding treasures in boxes.

◆ Large cardboard boxes in outdoor area – make into homes, castles, etc.

◆ Dough beside plastic boxes with lids – how much dough can you get in?

◆ Throw the beanbags/balls into the box.

◆ Obstacle course for children – avoid the boxes.

◆ Play tunnel made out of large boxes for children to crawl through and hide inside.

◆ Delivery games – can you take this box over to David? David take it to Zainab, etc …

Knowledge and understanding of the world

◆ *Activity plan: Tunnels and bridges made from boxes (p. 82)*

◆ Display: Presents – do you remember getting anything special in a box?

◆ Look at these boxes – what are they made of?

◆ Look at these plastic, wooden and paper boxes: What will happen if we put this selection of boxes in water?

◆ Can you make you a car or something to sit in out of this large box?

◆ Where can we see boxes in our environment?

◆ Old and new boxes – guess what they are used for?

◆ A small box of treasure is buried in the sand.

Mathematical development
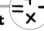

◆ *Activity plan: Teddy's button box (p. 80)*

◆ Sorting boxes – according to size.

◆ Sorting boxes – according to colour.

◆ How many teddy bears/cuddly toys can fit into this box?

◆ How many scoops of sand to fill up this small box?

◆ Predict how many buttons can fit into this box?

◆ Can you put these boxes inside each other?

◆ Can you make this box heavier than this other box?

◆ Which of these two boxes is the taller? Which is heavier?

◆ Lift the lid on the boxes – which one has three buttons in it?

1 A shoebox of memories

Have you any photographs or items that help you feel happy? Shall we put them in a special box for you?

Specific resources

- shoe box or similar box
- fabric
- pencils
- paper or other materials to be used as a lining for the box
- labels
- paint and materials to decorate the box

Key learning intentions

This activity will help children to talk about special events in their lives and encourage them to think positively about themselves and their family. It will also help children to build a relationship with an adult and develop their speaking skills.

Links to Foundation Stage curriculum		
Area of learning	**Aspects of learning**	**Curriculum guidance page**
Personal, social and emotional development	Disposition and attitudes Self-confidence and self-esteem Making relationships Behaviour and self-control Self-care Sense of community	32 34 36 38 40 42
Communication, language and literacy	Language for communication Language for thinking Reading Writing	48, 50, 52, 54 56–8 62 64
Mathematical development	Numbers as labels and for counting Calculating Shape, space and measures	74 76 78–80
Knowledge and understanding of the world	Exploration and investigation Designing and making skills Sense of time Sense of place Cultures and beliefs	86, 88 90 94 96 98
Physical development	Movement Using tools and materials	106, 108 114
Creative development	Exploring media and materials Imagination Responding to experiences, and expressing and communicating ideas	120 124 126

Ideas for organising the activity

This activity must be planned in advance as parents and carers should also be involved. It is important that children do not bring into your setting any items which have so much value that damage or loss would cause distress. Items such as photographs or small mementos will therefore work well. This activity should be carried out with individuals or pairs because it acts as a tool to help children talk about their feelings and their families.

Begin by looking at the items that children have brought. Can they tell you why they are special? Do they remember where they are from or when they had them? You can count the items with the child before thinking about choosing a box to fit them.

Ask the child to find a box and to choose the type of lining that they would like. Fabric, shredded paper or tissue paper would work well. Ask the child to decorate the box and also to 'write' their name or make a mark on a label so that it can be easily identified. Store the boxes safely – it may be a good idea to send them home at the end of the session.

Extending and varying children's learning

◆ Encourage children to show other children their items.
◆ Make your own box so that children can hear about your special memories.
◆ Encourage children to 'write' down or draw some of the memories.
◆ Show children other 'precious' items and ask them why special things are sometimes not 'shared'.

2 Guess what's in my box!

Look at these objects. Now listen to the sound I make when I shake the box. What's in the box?

Specific resources

◆ small boxes
◆ objects (that will fit in the box) made from different materials, e.g. metal spoons, fabric, pasta, buttons, shells, corks

---

Key learning intentions

This activity helps children's auditory discrimination skills, which will help them when they begin to read. It will also help children to experiment with sounds.

Links to Foundation Stage curriculum		
Area of learning	**Aspects of learning**	**Curriculum guidance page**
Personal, social and emotional development	Disposition and attitudes Self-confidence and self-esteem Making relationships Behaviour and self-control	32 34 36 38
Communication, language and literacy	Language for communication Language for thinking Linking sounds with letters	48, 50, 52, 54 56–8 60

Mathematical development	Numbers as labels and for counting Calculating Shape, space and measures	74 76 78–80
Knowledge and understanding of the world	Exploration and investigation	86, 88
Physical development	Movement Using tools and materials	106, 108 114
Creative development	Exploring media and materials Music	120 122

Ideas for organising the activity

This activity works well with small groups of children. Put out on a tray the objects that you intend to use (no more than ten). Encourage the children to feel and talk about them. Do they know what they are all used for, as well as their names? Count the objects.

Put one of the items into a box. Ask the children to guess which item is in the box. They take turns to shake the box. They can then take turns to hide objects in the box for the others to guess. If they are enjoying the game, you can have more than one box so that they work out which item is in which box!

Extending and varying children's learning

◆ Children can look for other objects around the room to play this game with.
◆ Ask the children to put the 'loudest' item in the box or the 'quietest'.
◆ Ask children to put their 'favourite' item in the box.
◆ Put out a selection of boxes with items in them on the interest table for children to play the game by themselves.
◆ Use three boxes with different items in – can they sort them by weight?

3 Teddy's button box

Teddy has lots of buttons. He wants to keep all his buttons together. Which of these boxes would be the best?

Specific resources

◆ 20–30 buttons
◆ three different sizes of boxes – one too small, one too large and one of good size
◆ pencil
◆ paper

> **Key learning intentions**
> This activity is designed to help children count, measure and problem solve.

Links to Foundation Stage curriculum		
Area of learning	**Aspects of learning**	**Curriculum guidance page**
Personal, social and emotional development	Disposition and attitudes Making relationships Self-care	32 36 40
Communication, language and literacy	Language for communication Language for thinking Writing	48, 50, 52, 54 56–8 64
Mathematical development	Numbers as labels and for counting Calculating Shape, space and measures	74 76 78–80
Knowledge and understanding of the world	Exploration and investigation	86, 88
Physical development	Movement Using tools and materials	106, 108 114
Creative development	Imagination	124

Ideas for organising the activity

This activity works well with pairs or individual children, so that they can be involved in the activity. Show the children teddy and tell them that teddy has some buttons. Encourage the children to talk about and explore the buttons. Which ones are their favourites? How many buttons are there?

Tell them teddy wants to find a box to put them in. He has brought along three different boxes. Which do they think will be the best box? Could they try them out? Use language such as 'smallest', 'smaller', 'larger' and 'largest'. Once the children

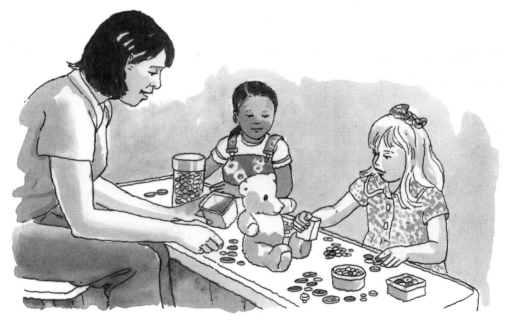

Teddy wants to find a box to put them in

have decided which is the best box, ask them if they could write a note to teddy to tell him which box he should keep his buttons in.

Extending and varying children's learning

◆ Leave teddy, the boxes and other objects out so that children can recreate this play.
◆ Reply to the children's letters on behalf of teddy so that children learn that writing is a way of communicating.
◆ Encourage the children to sort through the buttons and guess which ones are teddy's favourites.
◆ Ask the children if they would like to draw around the buttons.

4 Tunnels and bridges made from boxes

Can you make a tunnel out of these boxes so that the remote-controlled car can go through it or under it?

Specific resources

◆ sturdy boxes   ◆ scissors   ◆ paper
◆ pencils   ◆ remote-controlled car   ◆ stapler
◆ sticky tape

Key learning intentions
This activity is designed to help children use ICT and to develop their problem-solving skills.

Links to Foundation Stage curriculum

Area of learning	Aspects of learning	Curriculum guidance page
Personal, social and emotional development	Disposition and attitudes Making relationships Behaviour and self-control Self-care	32 36 38 40
Communication, language and literacy	Language for communication Language for thinking Writing	48, 50, 52, 54 56–8 64
Mathematical development	Numbers as labels and for counting Shape, space and measures	74 78–80
Knowledge and understanding of the world	Exploration and investigation Designing and making skills Information and communication technology	86, 88 90 92
Physical development	Sense of space Movement Using equipment Using tools and materials	104 106, 108 112 114

Creative development	Exploring media and materials	120
	Imagination	124
	Responding to experiences, and expressing and communicating ideas	126

Ideas for organising the activity

This activity works well with pairs of children. Begin by making sure that they have had time to play with the remote-controlled car. Make sure they understand how it works. Use this as an opportunity to model some positional language such as 'forwards', 'backwards', etc.

Put out the boxes and see if the children can make an obstacle course for the car. Develop this and see if children can think of ways of making bridges or tunnels for the car to travel through. This activity will require support from the adult, but try and make sure that the children are providing ideas and solutions. They will need plenty of time to develop their ideas. This activity also works well in an outdoor area.

Extending and varying children's learning

◆ Add in some small world toys so that children can elaborate their play and use their imagination.
◆ Ask children if they could draw a map to show where the tunnels and bridges have been placed.

5 Sandcastle boxes

Can you make sandcastles using these small boxes?

Specific resources

◆ play sand, either in small trays or in a large sand pit
◆ range of small boxes
◆ spoons
◆ cocktail sticks or straws
◆ labels
◆ paper
◆ pencils

> **Key learning intentions**
> This activity is designed to promote children's hand-eye co-ordination whilst giving them the opportunity to explore the properties of different sized boxes.

Links to Foundation Stage curriculum		
Area of learning	**Aspects of learning**	**Curriculum guidance page**
Personal, social and emotional development	Disposition and attitudes	32
	Behaviour and self-control	38
	Self-care	40
Communication, language and literacy	Language for communication	48, 50, 52, 54
	Language for thinking	56–8
	Writing	64

Mathematical development	Numbers as labels and for counting	74
	Calculating	76
	Shape, space and measures	78–80
Knowledge and understanding of the world	Exploration and investigation	86, 88
	Designing and making skills	90
	Information and communication technology	92
Physical development	Movement	106, 108
	Using tools and materials	114
Creative development	Exploring media and materials	120
	Imagination	124
	Responding to experiences, and expressing and communicating ideas	126

Ideas for organising the activity

This activity can be carried out with individual children or small groups. Sand can be put into a small tray such as a cat litter tray to allow several children to have their own sand.

Start by putting out a selection of small boxes in the sand tray or pit. Try out the boxes first to ensure that you have some that will make sandcastles! Ask the children if they could make a sandcastle using the boxes. Is it easier to use the boxes or beakers, or small buckets? Which boxes make the best sandcastles? Encourage children to make flags or decorate their sandcastles.

If they are successful at making box-shaped sandcastles, they may wish to use this as a backdrop, e.g. a village or town for small world play. Encourage them to tidy away after they have finished the activity. If possible, give them a hand-held vacuum cleaner to sweep up the sand so that they have the chance to operate equipment.

Extending and varying children's learning

◆ Can children make a small and a large sandcastle?
◆ Can they make a tunnel to go underneath the castle?
◆ Can they make a bridge to join two castles together?
◆ Can they hide something in their sandcastle?
◆ Read *Come Away from the Water, Shirley* by John Burningham.

6 Make a puppet theatre from a box

Would you like to make a puppet and a theatre for the puppet?

Specific resources

◆ wooden spoons   ◆ fabric   ◆ paint
◆ glue   ◆ shoebox

Key learning intentions
This activity will help children explore materials as well as use their imagination.

Links to Foundation Stage curriculum		
Area of learning	**Aspects of learning**	**Curriculum guidance page**
Personal, social and emotional development	Disposition and attitudes Making relationships Self-care	32 36 40
Communication, language and literacy	Language for communication Language for thinking	48, 50, 52, 54 56–8
Mathematical development	Shape, space and measures	78–80
Knowledge and understanding of the world	Exploration and investigation Designing and making skills	86, 88 90
Physical development	Movement Using tools and materials	106, 108 114
Creative development	Exploring media and materials Imagination Responding to experiences, and expressing and communicating ideas	120 124 126

Ideas for organising the activity

This activity works well with individual children or pairs, as most children will need adult support. Begin by showing children the wooden spoons. Show them how the flat rounded surface of the spoon could be made into a face and the handle decorated with fabric so that the spoon can be made into a puppet. Give children a wide range of choice of fabric, ribbons, lace and other materials to make clothes for their puppet. Wool or cotton wool can be used as hair. The key to this activity is to encourage children to make their own choices, so while showing them how to join or use materials, ensure that they are active in the process.

The shoebox theatre is easily made. The bottom of the box should be cut out, then children can paint or decorate it. This type of activity presents a wonderful opportunity for children to talk freely with an adult and can also be used to help children to count, measure and imagine the characters of their puppet.

Extending and varying children's learning

◆ Encourage older children to support younger children while making their puppets.
◆ Use spoon puppets as props for story telling.
◆ Ask children to talk to each other about their puppets.

Theme 5 Cars

Most children have been in a car: going in a car may be part of their everyday lives. Cars hold a fascination for children as they are seen as part of the adult world. As a starting point, 'cars' is a useful theme because it can be widened out to look at journeys, as well as other forms of transport such as boats, trains and buses.

Inside the box on each area of learning below is a range of ideas for activities and stories on the theme of cars. You will find on the following pages a ready-made activity plan for the first idea listed in each box. In addition, all the stories mentioned are listed in the Booklist on pages 250–252.

Ideas to suggest to parents

◆ Point out road signs and safe places to cross.

◆ Show their child the name of the road where they live.

◆ Point out the registration plates of different cars.

◆ Point out differences between cars, e.g. old, new, shiny, colour.

Personal, social and emotional development

◆ *Activity plan: The bus game (p. 88)*

◆ Visit by a lollipop person.

◆ Visit by a road safety officer.

◆ Tell me about a journey that you have taken.

◆ Here are some boxes – can you help each other to make a train or a bus?

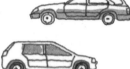
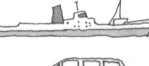
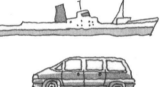
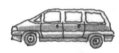
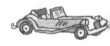

Communication, language and literacy

◆ *Activity plan: Role-play area: At the petrol station (p. 89)*

◆ Draw 'maps' or give instructions for teddy to move from one place to another in the setting.

◆ Rhymes and songs:
  ◆ 'Row, row, row your boat'
  ◆ 'Wheels on the bus'

◆ Stories:
  ◆ *Are We Nearly There?*
  ◆ *Here Comes the Train*
  ◆ *The Little Boat*
  ◆ *I Love Boats*
  ◆ *Mary's Secret*
  ◆ *My Puffer Train*
  ◆ *Trucks*

◆ Write registration plates for cars.

◆ Teddy has a new car – can you describe it?

◆ Look at all these toy cars – can you guess which one I am describing?

Creative development

- *Activity plan: Make a car for teddy's friend (p. 94)*
- Song and action rhymes:
  - 'Row, row, row your boat'
  - 'Wheels on the bus'
- Dip cars into a tray of paint – what tracks do they make?
- Construction toys – can you make a road layout?
- Drama – pretend you are a car – can you go fast, slow, in and out?
- Role-play area: Inside a car – complete with seats, maps, road atlases.
- Cars and vehicles with dough – what marks do they leave?

Physical development

- *Activity plan: Washing the tricycles and toys in the outdoor area (p. 93)*
- Chalk lines in the outdoor area – draw your own road with chalk.
- Pretend you are a car – can you go in and out of these cones?
- Dough and toy cars – can you make tyre prints?
- Car game – stop and go.
- Toy cars in the sand pit – make a road layout.

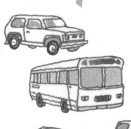
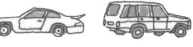
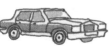
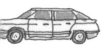

Knowledge and understanding of the world

- *Activity plan: Make a ferry for the toy cars (p. 91)*
- What do you go past on the way to the setting?
- Maps of the local area – which road do you live on?
- Display: Journeys we have taken.
- Remote-controlled cars – can you keep your car in this space?
- Toy cars and vehicles in the sand area.

Mathematical development

- *Activity plan: Measure how far your car can travel (p. 90)*
- How many cars in the feely bag: one, two, three or more?
- Sort toy cars, buses and lorries.
- Order toy cars into sizes.
- How many toy cars to balance this weight?
- Sort toy cars into colours, number of doors.
- Which box has the most cars in it?
- Make a bus or train for the small world people.

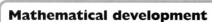

Activity plans for the theme 'cars'

I The bus game

Come and look at this fun game. Everyone starts with an empty bus and then we try to fill it up with children.

Specific resources

◆ prepared sheet with a simple outline of a double-decker bus with six square windows
◆ small photos of children (could be of the children themselves)
◆ dice with numbers 1 and 2 only
◆ glue

Key learning intentions

This activity helps children to take turns and build relationships.

Links to Foundation Stage curriculum		
Area of learning	**Aspects of learning**	**Curriculum guidance page**
Personal, social and emotional development	Disposition and attitudes Self-confidence and self-esteem Making relationships Self-care Sense of community	32 34 36 40 42
Communication, language and literacy	Language for communication Language for thinking Linking sounds with letters Reading Writing	48, 50, 52, 54 56–8 60 62 64
Knowledge and understanding of the world	Designing and making skills Sense of time	90 94
Physical development	Using equipment Using tools and materials	112 114
Creative development	Responding to experiences, and expressing and communicating ideas	126

Ideas for organising the activity

Prepare the bus sheets. Draw a simple outline of a double-decker bus (see opposite). Make sure there are three windows on the top deck and another three windows below. Prepare the dice by putting small stickers over the sides of the dice. Put either one or two dots on the stickers so that when children throw the dice they will only be able to throw a 1 or a 2.

Play this game with pairs or trios of children. This type of game is excellent for children who are finding it hard to socialise with others, as being close to an adult may give them the confidence to talk to other children. Give each child a bus sheet and six photos. Tell the children that they are drivers of the bus and when they throw

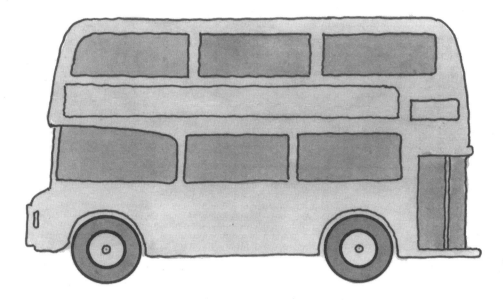

the dice they must take on the number of passengers shown on the dice. The children pick up the correct number of photos and stick each onto a blank square. When each bus is full, the game has come to an end. Afterwards, the buses can be displayed for everyone to see.

Use this game as a way of talking about how children get to the setting. Have they ever waited for a bus?

Extending and varying children's learning

- ◆ Increase the numbers of windows on the bus and the numbers shown on the dice.
- ◆ Encourage children to draw pictures of children in the windows on the bus.
- ◆ Play a variation of the game – the bus is full and the children empty the bus by taking off the pictures (these can be mounted on cards).

2 Role-play area: At the petrol station

Cars, ambulances, taxis and even buses need petrol to keep them going. What happens in a petrol station? What can you buy there?

Specific resources

- ◆ large cardboard boxes to act as petrol pumps
- ◆ cardboard boxes large enough for children to sit in to act as cars
- ◆ cash till   ◆ newspapers   ◆ small boxes
- ◆ area to act as shop   ◆ disposable gloves   ◆ buckets
- ◆ tools

> **Key learning intentions**
> This activity will help children to extend their vocabulary and encourage them to play alongside or with others.

Links to Foundation Stage curriculum		
Area of learning	**Aspects of learning**	**Curriculum guidance page**
Personal, social and emotional development	Disposition and attitudes	32
Communication, language and literacy	Language for communication Language for thinking Reading Writing	48, 50, 52, 54 56–8 62 64
Mathematical development	Numbers as labels and for counting Calculating Shape, space and measures	74 76 78–80
Knowledge and understanding of the world	Exploration and investigation Sense of place	86, 88 96
Physical development	Using tools and materials	114
Creative development	Exploring media and materials	120

Ideas for organising the activity

Talk to the children about what happens in a petrol station. Many children will have been inside the shop part, although they may not know what the pump is for. If possible, make sure parents know that this will be the theme for a role-play area so that they can talk to children if they have a car. As with any role play, children will gain more if an adult can spend some time modelling the language. Some petrol stations may be prepared to lend overalls and items such as disposable gloves to help the role play seem authentic. Encourage children to 'customise' their cars, e.g. paint, add stickers.

> **Health and safety**
> Take this opportunity to talk to children about the danger of walking around in petrol stations unsupervised or touching things in cars if ever they are left inside them.

Extending and varying children's learning

- Encourage children to make props for the petrol stations, e.g. newspapers and magazines, bags, bottles and boxes.
- Add a car wash section complete with sponges, wipes and buckets.

3 Measure how far your car can travel

Choose a car. Let it roll down the slope. How far does it travel? Which car will go the furthest?

Specific resources

- toy cars
- piece of stiff card or wood to make a ramp
- string, ribbons or other materials that children can use to measure with

Key learning intentions
This activity will help children learn about measuring and encourage the use of positional language.

Links to Foundation Stage curriculum		
Area of learning	**Aspects of learning**	**Curriculum guidance page**
Personal, social and emotional development	Disposition and attitudes Behaviour and self-control	32 38
Communication, language and literacy	Language for communication Language for thinking	48, 50, 52, 54 56–8
Mathematical development	Shape, space and measures	78–80
Knowledge and understanding of the world	Designing and making skills	90
Physical development	Sense of space Movement Using tools and materials	104 106, 108 114
Creative development	Exploring media and materials	120

Ideas for organising the activity

This activity works well with pairs of children or very small groups. Begin by encouraging the children to roll and play with the cars. Build a ramp using a stiff piece of card or wood propped up on some books or other items. Ask the children if they would like to see how far their car will roll.

Talk to the children about how they could measure the distance. Show them how ribbons or string could be used to measure from the starting point to the end point. Encourage them to see if they have any other ideas. They may, for example, count the number of steps that it takes to reach the car.

Use this activity as a way of encouraging children to think about how to make cars roll further, e.g. by adjusting the height of the slope.

Extending and varying children's learning

◆ What happens if the slope is put onto a carpet – do the cars still roll as far?
◆ Can the children match cars to words such as furthest, nearest?
◆ Can the children match cars to positions, e.g. first, second and third?
◆ Encourage children to roll other objects to see which ones go the furthest.

4 Make a ferry for the toy cars

Some special boats take cars on them so that people can go on holiday. They are called ferries. Have you ever been on a ferry?

Specific resources

- water tray
- paper
- scissors
- toy cars
- pencils
- plastic containers, e.g. margarine tubs and lids
- play people
- glue
- photos of ferries from magazines or travel brochures

Key learning intentions

This activity should help children's problem solving, and designing and making skills.

Links to Foundation Stage curriculum

Area of learning	Aspects of learning	Curriculum guidance page
Personal, social and emotional development	Disposition and attitudes	32
Communication, language and literacy	Language for communication Language for thinking Linking sounds with letters Reading Writing	48, 50, 52, 54 56–8 60 62 64
Mathematical development	Shape, space and measures	78–80
Knowledge and understanding of the world	Sense of time	94
Physical development	Using tools and materials	114
Creative development	Responding to experiences, and expressing and communicating ideas	126

Ideas for organising the activity

This activity works well with small groups of children or pairs. Begin by asking if any of the children have been on a ferry – this will vary from setting to setting. Show photos of ferries for children to understand what a ferry does.

Show how a car will normally sink in the water. Ask the children if they could make a boat or find a way of moving the car safely across the water tray. For younger children this may mean just putting a car inside a margarine tub, whilst for older children it may mean spending time customising materials.

Use this as an opportunity for children to talk about different ways in which they have travelled. Some children will have been on an aeroplane whilst others will have been on trains, buses and trams. Aim to model specific vocabulary such as 'launch', 'load', 'crossing', 'journey' and 'vessel'.

Extending and varying children's learning

- Create a dock scene in the water tray using boats, lorries, ticket offices, etc.
- Encourage children to produce 'tickets' for the cars to travel on the ferry.
- Use play people to accompany the cars on board.
- Encourage children to make a collage of photos of different types of boats, ferries and other seacraft.

5 Washing the tricycles and toys in the outdoor area

Would you like to wash the toys outside? What will we need?

Specific resources

- buckets
- sponges
- soapy warm water
- protective clothing

Key learning intentions
The aim of this activity is to strengthen children's arm muscles and develop gross motor movements.

Links to Foundation Stage curriculum		
Area of learning	**Aspects of learning**	**Curriculum guidance page**
Personal, social and emotional development	Disposition and attitudes Self-confidence and self-esteem Making relationships Behaviour and self-control Self-care	32 34 36 38 40
Communication, language and literacy	Language for communication Language for thinking Reading Writing Handwriting	48, 50, 52, 54 56–8 62 64 66
Mathematical development	Numbers as labels and for counting	74

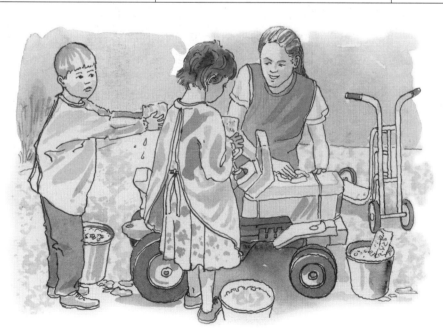

Warm water is always a success!

Knowledge and understanding of the world	Exploration and investigation	86, 88
Physical development	Sense of space	104
	Health and bodily awareness	110
	Using equipment	112
	Using tools and materials	114
Creative development	Imagination	124
	Responding to experiences, and expressing and communicating ideas	126

Ideas for organising the activity

This activity works best with small groups of children or pairs. Children enjoy helping and washing with sponges, and warm water is always a success. Some water on clothes is almost inevitable, so parents should be warned that spare clothes may be needed. Take out some of the larger equipment that children can wipe and wash safely. Model language to the children during the washing, such as 'squeeze', 'wipe', 'drip', 'foam', 'bubbles'.

Use this activity to talk about the importance of keeping things clean and tidy as part of caring for the environment. When the children have finished, make sure they wash and rinse their hands thoroughly to avoid any skin irritation. Take photos of the children as they are washing.

Health and safety
This activity needs to be carefully planned. Children with sensitive skin may need to wear protective gloves. Choose objects for washing that will not trap children's fingers. As with any activity involving water, children must be closely supervised.

Extending and varying the activity

◆ If possible take children to a real car wash!
◆ Read books about washing such as *The Wild Washerwomen*.
◆ Encourage children to talk about things that are washed in their homes, e.g. dishes, clothes.
◆ Watch how long it takes for the puddles in the outside area to 'disappear'.

6 Make a car for teddy's friend

Here is teddy's friend. Teddy wonders if you could make a car for him.

Specific resources

◆ assorted sizes of boxes
◆ paint
◆ glue
◆ sticky tape
◆ other junk modelling materials

◆ CD-ROMS (good to act as wheels)
◆ crayons
◆ stapler
◆ clingfilm

Key learning intentions
This activity will help children to choose materials independently and encourage their designing and making skills.

Links to Foundation Stage curriculum		
Area of learning	**Aspects of learning**	**Curriculum guidance page**
Personal, social and emotional development	Disposition and attitudes Self-confidence and self-esteem Self-care	32 34 40
Communication, language and literacy	Language for communication Language for thinking Linking sounds with letters Reading Writing	48, 50, 52, 54 56–8 60 62 64
Mathematical development	Shape, space and measures	78–80
Knowledge and understanding of the world	Exploration and investigation Designing and making skills Information and communication technology	86, 88 90 92
Physical development	Using equipment Using tools and materials	112 114
Creative development	Exploring media and materials Imagination Responding to experiences, and expressing and communicating ideas	120 124 126

Ideas for organising the activity

This activity is ideal for pairs of children or small groups. Large groups tend to be less practicable as children will require support and adult attention. Begin by showing teddy's friend to the children. This can be a cuddly toy of any size. Tell the children that he would like a car or something that he can travel in. Encourage them to ask teddy questions – Why does he need a car? What type of car? Does his friend have a favourite colour? These questions may need to be modelled for the children.

   Show children the materials available. Encourage them to plan a little and to keep checking that teddy's friend will fit into the vehicle! This will help them with their measuring skills. Do not worry if the vehicles look original – the aim of this activity is to encourage children to explore materials rather than to make a car to a set design.

Extending and varying children's learning

◆ Teddy's friend sends the children a thank-you letter.
◆ Children 'write' to teddy about how to use the 'car' safely.
◆ Photos are taken of the cars with teddy's friend inside.
◆ Children make cars from other construction equipment, e.g. Duplo.
◆ Children make a boat for teddy's friend.
◆ Children use their cars in the sand area.

Theme 6 Clothes

This theme provides a good starting point as all children wear clothes and often notice the clothes that they are wearing. Clothes are also very personal to children and their families, so opportunities can be taken for children to share with other children clothes that have special meaning for them or their families.

Inside the box on each area of learning below is a range of ideas for activities and stories on the theme of clothes. You will find on the following pages a ready-made activity plan for the first idea listed in each box. In addition, all the stories mentioned are listed in the Booklist on pages 250–252.

Ideas to suggest to parents

◆ Encourage their child to get dressed and to choose appropriate clothes.

◆ Point out how clothes fasten.

◆ Talk to their child about clothes that are important in their family, e.g. christening robes, wedding outfits.

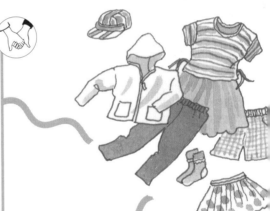

Personal, social and emotional development

◆ Activity plan: *Can we pack a case for teddy?* (p. 98)

◆ Display: My favourite clothes.

◆ Hanging up and sorting out the dressing-up clothes.

◆ Favourite clothes – which of these do you like best?

◆ Clothes that make you feel good.

◆ Teddy doesn't want to put a coat on – can you explain to him why he needs to?

◆ Can you help each other to find your pegs and hang up your coats?

Communication, language and literacy

◆ Activity plan: *Whose shoes?* (p. 99)

◆ Stories:
  ◆ *Doing the Washing*
  ◆ *New Shoes for Silvia*
  ◆ *Sloth's Shoes*
  ◆ *Two Shoes, New Shoes*
  ◆ *The Wild Washerwomen*

◆ Role-play area: Shoe shop, the Odd shop (where nothing matches!)

◆ Story bag: Guess what has teddy been doing? – He has these clothes in his bag!

◆ Feely bag: What types of clothes are in this bag?

◆ Welcome to our shoe shop.

◆ Sequence cards – getting dressed.

Creative development

- *Activity plan: Button, fabric and lace collage (p. 104)*
- Can you make a colour to match your jumper, shoes or this scarf?
- Button rubbings.
- Writing and drawing with fabric crayons on T-shirts.
- Role-play area: Clothes shop.
- Choose some shoes – decide how you would walk in them if they were yours.
- Move to the music – what would you like to dress up in?

Physical development

- *Activity plan: Dancing and moving to music with scarves and ribbons (p. 102)*
- Hanging out washing on a line to dry.
- Folding sheets and blankets.
- Parachute games using items of clothing.
- Welly throwing.
- Which of these clothes would you need to keep warm on a cold day?
- Buttons with dough.
- Find the buttons in the sand pit.

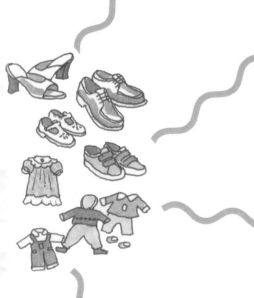

Knowledge and understanding of the world

- *Activity plan: Can we dress teddy? (p. 101)*
- Which of these clothes will dry quickest?
- Display: Special clothes, clothes for celebrations: I remember wearing these clothes when …
- Who wears these clothes?
- Clothes I have grown out of – encourage children to bring in and talk about them.
- Clothes for different times of the year – match the clothes to the weather!
- Fabrics – which of these fabrics feels the softest?
- Can you sew on buttons?

Mathematical development

- *Activity plan: Button patterns (p. 100)*
- Sorting clothes by one feature, e.g. colour, type, with buttons, fabric.
- Ordering clothes according to size.
- Pairs, e.g. gloves, mittens, socks, shoes.
- How many buttons in the feely bag?
- How many buttons can fit into this small box?
- Weighing clothes, e.g. find clothes that are as heavy as this towel.
- Compare shoes – which one is the largest?
- Sort gloves – what are the different types used for?

Activity plans for the theme 'clothes'

I Can we pack a case for teddy?

Teddy's going on holiday for two days. Can we pack a suitcase for him so that everything fits?

Specific resources

◆ small box or suitcase
◆ clothes

◆ items such as toothbrush
  ◆ soap
  ◆ towel
  ◆ facecloth

Key learning intentions
This activity will help children to practise their self-help skills, think about the importance of personal hygiene and develop their language for communication and thinking. Children should also be encouraged to think about how many things teddy will need.

Links to Foundation Stage curriculum

Area of learning	Aspects of learning	Curriculum guidance page
Personal, social and emotional development	Disposition and attitudes Making relationships Behaviour and self-control Self-care	32 36 38 40
Communication, language and literacy	Language for communication Language for thinking	48, 50, 52, 54 56–8
Mathematical development	Numbers as labels and for counting Calculating Shape, space and measures	74 76 78–80
Knowledge and understanding of the world	Exploration and investigation	86, 88
Physical development	Using tools and materials	114

Ideas for organising the activity

This activity can be carried out in pairs or small groups (no more than four or five) so that children can talk spontaneously. Start by bringing in teddy and an overflowing suitcase.

Some children may remember going on holiday. Let them look at all the items and name them so that they are hearing specific vocabulary. Ask them to work out what they think each item is for and which ones teddy will definitely need. Ask them to tell teddy what they are going to pack for him. Focus on the items required for personal hygiene, e.g. toothbrush, soap and hairbrush.

Using teddy as a stooge, pretend that he wants to take something that is not required. Ask the children to tell him why he cannot take it.

Extending and varying children's learning

◆ Read stories about going on holiday.
◆ Ask children to telephone teddy's mum to tell him that he is now packed.
◆ Encourage the children to write to teddy's mum to let her know what they have packed.
◆ Ask the children to write a luggage label for teddy's suitcase.
◆ Encourage teddy to send a letter or postcard to the children.

2 Whose shoes?

Let's look and see what is in these shoeboxes. Who do you think these shoes may belong to?

Specific resources

◆ shoeboxes filled with a range of footwear, e.g. slippers, men's shoes, baby shoes (where possible shoes should be selected that have special meaning for the children in your group, e.g. bridesmaid shoes or favourite slippers)

Key learning intentions
This activity is designed to promote children's overall language development, concentrating particularly on descriptive language and language for explaining.

Links to Foundation Stage curriculum

Area of learning	Aspects of learning	Curriculum guidance page
Personal, social and emotional development	Disposition and attitudes Sense of community	32 42
Communication, language and literacy	Language for communication Language for thinking	48, 50, 52, 54 56–8
Mathematical development	Numbers as labels and for counting Shape, space and measures	74 78–80
Knowledge and understanding of the world	Sense of time Cultures and beliefs	94 98
Physical development	Using tools and materials	114

Ideas for organising the activity

Show small groups or individual children several shoeboxes. Ask them if they would like to open a box and see what is inside. Can they guess what the shoes are used for? What do they look like? Who do the children think used them? Do they recognise the shoes? If possible, include footwear that will have special meaning for the children you are working with. This will help them to use language to explain and also recall.

The activity should also include opportunities for children to count the boxes and also to find the largest pair of shoes. This may be a good starting point for children before putting the shoes in a role-play area.

Health and safety
Make sure that shoes are clean.

Extending and varying children's learning

◆ Ask the children to choose their favourite pair of shoes.
◆ Encourage the children to draw or 'write' about their favourite shoes.
◆ Ask the children to sort shoes into colours or types.
◆ Play games such as 'giant's footsteps'.

3 Button patterns

Look at this line of buttons. Can you see the pattern that I am making?

Specific resources

◆ 'real' buttons so that children can enjoy the textures

Key learning intentions
The aim of this activity is to focus children on spotting simple patterns and working out how to add to a pattern. Sorting skills are used in order for children to continue a pattern. Children should also practise their skills of explaining their rationale for adding to a pattern.

Links to Foundation Stage curriculum		
Area of learning	**Aspects of learning**	**Curriculum guidance page**
Personal, social and emotional development	Disposition and attitudes	32
Communication, language and literacy	Language for communication Language for thinking	48, 50, 52, 54 56–8
Mathematical development	Numbers as labels and for counting	74
Knowledge and understanding of the world	Exploration and investigation	86, 88
Physical development	Using tools and materials	114
Creative development	Exploring materials and media	120

Ideas for organising the activity

'Real' buttons have a magical appeal for children and should be put out regularly for children to play with and explore. This activity can be carried out with individuals or pairs. Encourage them to 'play' with the buttons before showing them simple patterns.

Look for ways of helping children to describe and explain their rationale for adding to a pattern. If they lack the specific language skills, consider using a stooge such as a puppet or teddy, and model the language by explaining the pattern to the stooge.

Children who cannot 'see' the pattern should be encouraged to match or sort buttons. This activity is an ideal vehicle for a variety of naturalistic assessments such as counting, matching and sorting.

Extending and varying children's learning

◆ Can children produce large, small, large, small patterns?
◆ Can children add to a pattern based on the number of holes a button has?
◆ Can children add to a pattern based on whether buttons can roll?
◆ Ask children to make up their own 'colour' pattern.
◆ Ask children to draw around the buttons or do a rubbing with them.
◆ Ask children to sort out their favourite buttons to show teddy.
◆ Using teddy as a stooge, ask the children if they can write a note to his mum about his favourite buttons.

4 Can we dress teddy?

Teddy is hoping that you can make him something to wear. What would you like to make him? A hat, a scarf, or just something to put around him?

Specific resources

◆ teddy or small cuddly toy
◆ wide range of materials, e.g. paper, fabric, ribbons, scarves, card, crayons

> **Key learning intentions**
> This activity is to help children design and make something for teddy. The result is not as important as the process and the enjoyment of the children in having a go! Communication can also be a focus of this activity – children should be encouraged to ask questions about what teddy would like.

Links to Foundation Stage curriculum		
Area of learning	**Aspects of learning**	**Curriculum guidance page**
Personal, social and emotional development	Disposition and attitudes Self-care	32 40
Communication, language and literacy	Language for communication Language for thinking	48, 50, 52, 54 56–8
Mathematical development	Shape, space and measures	78–80
Knowledge and understanding of the world	Exploration and investigation Designing and making skills	86, 88 90
Physical development	Using equipment Using tools and materials	112 114
Creative development	Exploring media and materials	120

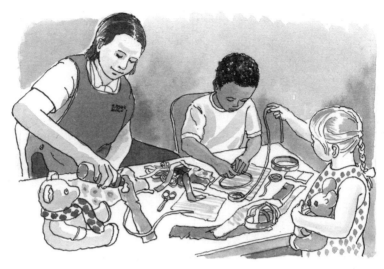

Make it clear that teddy is very easily satisfied!

Ideas for organising the activity

Using a teddy or similar stooge, tell a child or small group of children that teddy has asked if they could make him something to wear. Model some questions to ask teddy about what he likes and wants. Encourage the children to ask him questions, e.g. 'Do you like red?' Make it clear to them that teddy is very easily satisfied!

The key to this activity is encouraging children to be as independent as possible in design and making. Be supportive rather than directive: allow them to make mistakes, but help them consider ways of moving forward. Some very young children will simply stick something over teddy's head, while others may make quite a project of it. It is essential that teddy says 'thank you' and seems delighted with his new wardrobe.

Extending and varying children's learning

◆ Teddy writes a note of thanks to each child.
◆ Ask the children to make a specific item, e.g. a hat or a tunic.
◆ Encourage the children to try some simple sewing, using binker fabric.
◆ Make a collage showing teddy a range of clothes that he might like to wear.

5 Dancing and moving to music with scarves and ribbons

Look at all these lovely ribbons and scarves. Can you wave them in the air? Can you make large circles with them?

Specific resources

◆ scarves   ◆ ribbons   ◆ music

Key learning intentions

This activity is designed to promote children's physical development, especially gross motor co-ordination. The development of these physical skills will also help children develop the good hand-eye co-ordination that is later necessary for fluent handwriting.

Links to Foundation Stage curriculum

Area of learning	Aspects of learning	Curriculum guidance page
Personal, social and emotional development	Disposition and attitudes Behaviour and self-control	32 38
Communication, language and literacy	Language for thinking Handwriting	56–8 66
Mathematical development	Shape, space and measures	78–80
Knowledge and understanding of the world	Exploration and investigation	86, 88
Physical development	Sense of space Movement	104 106, 108
Creative development	Music	122

Ideas for organising the activity

Put out a selection of scarves and ribbons for children to choose. If possible, have sufficient amounts so that they can have an item in each hand. To make this activity as creative as possible, encourage children to make their own shapes and movements in the air. Introduce new vocabulary into the activity by providing a 'running commentary', e.g. 'Well done, you managed to *flick* the ribbon high into the air.'

Once the children have enjoyed making their own shapes and movements, you may wish to play some music so that they can move to the music.

Health and safety

To avoid ribbons being flicked into eyes, do not provide very long ribbons. This activity will need supervising in case children decide to put ribbons around necks!

Extending and varying children's learning

◆ Play 'follow my leader' type games with the scarves.
◆ Play games where children make circles by holding scarves or ribbons.
◆ Tie some simple knots in the scarves and encourage children to undo them.
◆ Make wind mobiles using the ribbons.
◆ Use the ribbons outdoors in windy weather.

6 Button, fabric and lace collage

Look at all these lovely things that are usually put onto clothes. Would you like to play and stick with them?

Specific resources

- pictures of clothes
- stiff paper
- as much haberdashery as possible, e.g. buttons, lace, feathers, sequins, beads, ribbons
- glue
- scissors

Key learning intentions

This activity aims to encourage children to learn specific vocabulary in relation to clothes, and also to explore the texture, shapes and colours of the items.

Links to Foundation Stage curriculum

Area of learning	Aspects of learning	Curriculum guidance page
Personal, social and emotional development	Disposition and attitudes Self-care	32 40
Communication, language and literacy	Language for communication Language for thinking	48, 50, 52, 54 56–8
Mathematical development	Shape, space and measures	78–80
Knowledge and understanding of the world	Exploration and investigation Designing and making skills	86, 88 90
Physical development	Using equipment Using tools and materials	112 114
Creative development	Exploring media and materials Responding to experiences, and expressing and communicating ideas	120 126

Ideas for organising the activity

The key to this activity is the appeal of the different items that children can touch, cut and stick. Magazines with pictures of clothes can also be used, but where possible the focus should be on the items of haberdashery. As children touch and hold items, name the items for them so that they absorb the new vocabulary. Some children will randomly stick, while others may be keen to produce a pattern or develop their own focus such as colour. Listening to children's rationale for their choices of materials will be interesting.

Health and safety

Supervise small items such as beads and sequins carefully, especially if the setting also has children under three years.

Extending and varying children's learning

◆ Encourage children to combine media, e.g. paint, then add collage.
◆ Encourage some children to try decorating garments used in the role-play area, e.g. sew on buttons, glue on sequins.
◆ Use some of the materials for children to print with.
◆ Use fabric as the background for the collage rather than paper.

Theme 7 Friends

This is a wonderful theme because most children from around three years of age are beginning to develop friendships. The theme lends itself particularly well to delivering the personal, social and emotional development area of learning. It can be used as a starting-point for looking at celebrations, families and people who help us.

Inside the box on each area of learning below is a range of ideas for activities and stories on the theme of friends. You will find on the following pages a ready-made activity plan for the first idea listed in each box. In addition, all the stories mentioned are listed in the Booklist on pages 250–252.

Ideas to suggest to parents
- ◆ Talk to their child about their own childhood friends.
- ◆ Help their child to phone a friend.
- ◆ Look at photos of their friends with their child.

Personal, social and emotional development
- ◆ *Activity plan: Display: We're all different, we're all special! (p. 108)*
- ◆ What makes you laugh? Can you make me laugh?
- ◆ Bring in photos of your friends and people who are special.
- ◆ Follow my friend (played like 'follow my leader').
- ◆ Who do you enjoy playing and being with?
- ◆ Choose a game to play with your friend – find out which one he or she would like best.

Communication, language and literacy
- ◆ *Activity plan: Write a letter to your friend (p. 109)*
- ◆ Stories:
  - ◆ *Elephant and Crocodile*
  - ◆ *Elmer*
  - ◆ *Mr Gumpy's Outing*
- ◆ Can you follow your friend's chalk lines on the ground?
- ◆ Name treasure hunt – can you recognise your friend's name?
- ◆ I am describing one of the children here today – can you guess whom?
- ◆ Ask your friend which of these is their favourite toy?
- ◆ Hide this object – can you tell your friend how to find it?
- ◆ Find the object that begins with the same letter of your friend's name.
- ◆ Describe a photo to your friends – can they guess which one you are talking about?

Creative development

- *Activity plan: Let's make our own patchwork (p. 115)*
- Can you mix paint to match the colour of your friend's jumper or top?
- Let's make up songs about the names of your friends.
- Role play area – invite your friends for tea.
- Look at these lovely clothes, shoes and hats – can you dress your friend up?
- Come and do a huge painting with your friend.
- Using photos of your friends – can you make a collage picture?

Physical development

- *Activity plan: Mud play: Can we hide our hands? (p. 113)*
- Let's play hide-and-seek with your friend.
- Dough – can you make cakes, sausages and chapattis for your friends?
- Play a game – one of you makes a print in the sand, the other guesses what they made it with.
- Can you throw a beanbag into the hoop where your friend is standing?

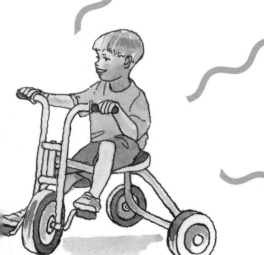

Knowledge and understanding of the world

- *Activity plan: Make a friendship bracelet (p. 111)*
- Display: Where do we meet our friends?
- Display: Fancy dress and celebrations we have been to.
- Can you use the computer to draw a picture for a friend?
- Bring in photos of your friends. Can you remember what you were doing?
- Come and take a photo of your friend.
- Let's make about a book about special days for your families.

Mathematical development

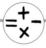

- *Activity plan: Mr Gumpy's boat game (p. 110)*
- Make a pattern with these buttons – can your friend copy it?
- Can you help teddy share these buttons with his two friends?
- Can you draw around your friend's hands? Which of you has the biggest hands?
- Your friend rolls the dice. Fill up your beaker with the number of scoops of sand shown on the dice.
- Put one, two or three objects in a bag – can your friend guess how many there are?

Activity plans for the theme 'friends'

I We're all different, we're all special!

Everyone is a little different and our friends are special because they are different. Let's look at the things that make you different and special!

Specific resources

◆ paper   ◆ crayons   ◆ photographs   ◆ pens
◆ markers   ◆ catalogues   ◆ mirrors

Key learning intentions
This activity will help children to think about the differences between us that make us special. It will help them consider their own unique identity.

Links to Foundation Stage curriculum

Area of learning	Aspects of learning	Curriculum guidance page
Personal, social and emotional development	Disposition and attitudes Self-confidence and self-esteem Making relationships Behaviour and self-control Self-care Sense of community	32 34 36 38 40 42
Communication, language and literacy	Language for communication Language for thinking Reading Writing Handwriting	48, 50, 52, 54 56–8 62 64 66
Mathematical development	Shape, space and measures	78–80
Knowledge and understanding of the world	Exploration and investigation Designing and making skills Cultures and beliefs	86, 88 90 98
Physical development	Movement Using equipment Using tools and materials	106, 108 112 114
Creative development	Exploring media and materials Responding to experiences, and expressing and communicating ideas	120 126

Ideas for organising the activity

This activity will need to be planned in advance so that children can bring in items or photographs if they wish. It works best with pairs or groups of about four so that each child can easily talk about their feelings and their families.

Begin by talking about how friends are special and often different. You might like to read the story of *Elmer* by David McKee as this looks at differences and friendships. Can they look at themselves in the mirror? Can they see ways in which they are different to each other – colour of eyes, number of teeth, etc? Can they think about other things that make them special – their favourite foods, the way in which they smile or laugh?

Once children have thought about what makes them different, encourage them to draw, cut out pictures or 'write' something towards a display. This should be an opportunity for children to learn that people are different and these differences should be valued.

Extending and varying children's learning

◆ Encourage children to say something that they like about each other.
◆ Encourage children to bring in a photo of someone special to them.
◆ Take photographs of children in the setting and use them to make children feel special.

2 Write a letter to your friend

Everyone likes to get a letter. Would you like to write a letter to your friend?

Specific resources

◆ writing paper
◆ pencils
◆ envelopes
◆ stamps
◆ markers
◆ crayons
◆ pens

Key learning intentions
This activity is designed to encourage children to make marks and to enjoy 'writing'.

Links to Foundation Stage curriculum		
Area of learning	**Aspects of learning**	**Curriculum guidance page**
Personal, social and emotional development	Disposition and attitudes	32
Communication, language and literacy	Language for communication Language for thinking Linking sounds with letters Reading Writing Handwriting	48, 50, 52, 54 56–8 60 62 64 66
Mathematical development	Shape, space and measures	78–80
Physical development	Movement Using tools and materials	106, 108 114
Creative development	Imagination Responding to experiences, and expressing and communicating ideas	124 126

Ideas for organising the activity

This activity works well with small groups of up to five children. Begin by asking children if they enjoy getting letters. You may wish to show the children some letters. Ask the children if they wish to send a letter to their friends.

Show the children the writing materials that are available – it is important that these are attractive and 'exciting'. Put out 'adult' pens, for example, so that children are tempted to use them. Tell the children that friends do not mind getting letters that they can't read and that they can always tell their friend what is in the letter. This prevents them becoming worried about their ability to 'write' properly. They may also want to send their friend a drawing or painting. Encourage them to put their letters in envelopes. They can also put a stamp on their letter.

Extending and varying children's learning

◆ Make a post box for letters.
◆ Encourage the children to make their own envelopes.
◆ Ask children to make a stamp for the letter.

3 Mr Gumpy's boat game

Do you remember that Mr Gumpy let his friends come on a boat ride?

Specific resources

◆ water tray
◆ farm animals

◆ boat or plastic container that will float
◆ dice

Key learning intentions
This activity will help children to count and recognise numbers.

Links to Foundation Stage curriculum

Area of learning	Aspects of learning	Curriculum guidance page
Personal, social and emotional development	Disposition and attitudes Self-confidence and self-esteem Making relationships Behaviour and self-control Self-care Sense of community	32 34 36 38 40 42
Communication, language and literacy	Language for communication Language for thinking	48, 50, 52, 54 56–8
Mathematical development	Numbers as labels and for counting Calculating Shape, space and measures	74 76 78–80
Physical development	Movement Using tools and materials	106, 108 114
Creative development	Imagination	124

Ideas for organising the activity

This activity works well with a small group of children. Begin by reading the book, *Mr Gumpy's Outing*. Ask the children to think about how the animals joined the boat. How many animals altogether went in his boat? Put out the plastic container or boat and the animals. Encourage the children to play with the animals by putting them in and out of the boat. How many animals will the boat take until it capsizes or sinks? Ask the children if they would like to play a game with a dice. One child rolls the dice and puts into the boat the number of animals shown on the dice. The children keep on adding animals until the boat sinks or capsizes. The dice can be altered to limit the number of digits e.g. the dice only shows a 1 or a 2.

Extending and varying children's learning

◆ Repeat this activity using different vessels – which one will hold the most animals?
◆ Play the game with the boat full – who can empty the boat first?
◆ Encourage the children to make their own boats to take the animals.

4 Make a friendship bracelet

Would you like to make a bracelet for your friend?

Specific resources

◆ beads   ◆ laces   ◆ dry pasta, which can be threaded, e.g. macaroni, penne
◆ pencils   ◆ paper   ◆ stapler
◆ glue   ◆ crayons

Key learning intentions
This activity is designed for children to explore materials and enjoy making a bracelet. It will also promote children's fine motor skills.

Links to Foundation Stage curriculum		
Area of learning	**Aspects of learning**	**Curriculum guidance page**
Personal, social and emotional development	Disposition and attitudes Self-confidence and self-esteem Making relationships Behaviour and self-control Self-care Sense of community	32 34 36 38 40 42
Communication, language and literacy	Language for communication Language for thinking Writing	48, 50, 52, 54 56–8 64
Mathematical development	Shape, space and measures	78–80

▽

Knowledge and understanding of the world	Exploration and investigation Designing and making skills Cultures and beliefs	86, 88 90 98
Physical development	Movement Using tools and materials	106, 108 114
Creative development	Exploring media and materials Responding to experiences, and expressing and communicating ideas	120 126

Ideas for organising the activity

This activity works well with small groups, or individual children if their physical skills are less developed. Begin by asking children if they have any special friends or people in their lives. Encourage them to talk about why they like being with some people – are they fun to play with or do they help them?

Tell the children that with the pasta, beads and laces we can make friendship bracelets or even necklaces. Encourage them to choose shapes they think are interesting. Some children may be ready to make patterns, while others will just want to thread. Ask them to think about the size of their bracelet – if it is too big, it will fall off the wrist. Can they think of ways of attaching the bracelet? (You may have to support them by showing them how to make a loop.) Ask them if they would like to think of ways to wrap up their bracelets – they could make envelopes or cards – or they may like to keep the bracelets themselves (in this case, maybe they could make one for themselves and another for a friend!).

Use this activity to help children to explore materials and their ideas. Avoid over-directing – the aim is to encourage children to make their own choices. You may also help children to talk about ways in which their family values special people.

Extending and varying children's learning

◆ Children can bring in or take photographs of their friends.
◆ Read the story *Aldo* about a child who has a special friend.
◆ Produce a display – 'Friends make me smile' – children can draw their friends.
◆ Play threading games – roll a dice and put on the number of beads shown.
◆ Can children copy a simple pattern that has been threaded onto a bracelet?

5 Mud play: Can we hide your friend's hands?

Let's make a mixture and see if you can hide your friend's hands and even these plastic animals.

Specific resources

◆ buckets   ◆ a range of spoons   ◆ water   ◆ sand
◆ mud   ◆ nail brush for washing hands afterwards

Key learning intentions
This activity is designed so that children can enjoy playing with natural materials outdoors. It also helps children to see the importance of hand washing.

Links to Foundation Stage curriculum		
Area of learning	**Aspects of learning**	**Curriculum guidance page**
Personal, social and emotional development	Disposition and attitudes Self-confidence and self-esteem Making relationships Behaviour and self-control Self-care	32 34 36 38 40
Communication, language and literacy	Language for communication Language for thinking Handwriting	48, 50, 52, 54 56–8 66
Knowledge and understanding of the world	Exploration and investigation Designing and making skills	86, 88 90
Physical development	Sense of space Movement Health and bodily awareness Using equipment Using tools and materials	104 106, 108 110 112 114
Creative development	Exploring media and materials Imagination Responding to experiences, and expressing and communicating ideas	120 124 126

Ideas for organising the activity

This activity works well with pairs of children or groups of up to four. Good supervision is necessary. Prepare for this activity by looking at your outdoor area and what might be suitable materials for children to use, e.g. grass, mud etc. You can either pick these materials and lay them out for the children or supervise the children as they gather them later.

Ask the children to put on protective clothes, to choose a bucket and spoon and come outdoors. Tell them that they can use sand, water and mud to make their own mixture. Afterwards they can put their hands into their 'muddy water'. Can they see their friend's hands? Encourage children to enjoy experimenting with their mixture – this is recreating a traditional type of play that many children used to play in their own homes.

Once children have finished playing, encourage them to rinse out their buckets before washing their hands thoroughly. Use nail brushes to clean under the nails. Use this activity as an opportunity to model language about how mud and water feels.

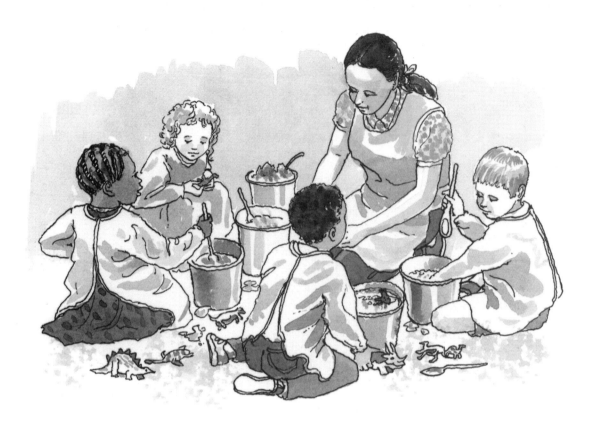

Encourage children to enjoy experimenting

Health and safety
This activity needs to be supervised and children need to know what they can and cannot put in their buckets.
  Once the activity has finished, children need to wash their hands thoroughly.

Extending and varying children's learning

◆ Ask children to hide other things in their mixture.
◆ Use a large tray outdoors. Can children model a scene, e.g. an island in the middle of a lake using the water, sand and mud?
◆ Encourage children to combine this type of play with their role play, e.g. this could be 'cooking'.
◆ Teach children the song 'Mud, Mud, Glorious Mud'.
◆ Ask children if they can bury each other's hands in the sand tray.

6 Let's make our own patchwork

In the book *Elmer*, the other elephants have an Elmer day to celebrate their friendship with him. They all become made of patchwork like him.

Specific resources

- fabrics – these could be brought from home
- glue
- stiff piece of card
- fabric scissors
- the book *Elmer*, by David McKee (see Booklist, pages 250–252)

Key learning intentions
This activity will help children explore materials and help them to feel part of a group.

Links to Foundation Stage curriculum		
Area of learning	**Aspects of learning**	**Curriculum guidance page**
Personal, social and emotional development	Disposition and attitudes Self-confidence and self-esteem Making relationships Behaviour and self-control Self-care Sense of community	32 34 36 38 40 42
Communication, language and literacy	Language for communication Language for thinking Reading Writing Handwriting	48, 50, 52, 54 56–8 62 64 66
Mathematical development	Shape, space and measures	78–80
Knowledge and understanding of the world	Exploration and investigation Designing and making skills Sense of time Sense of place Cultures and beliefs	86, 88 90 94 96 98
Physical development	Movement Using equipment Using tools and materials	106, 108 112 114
Creative development	Exploring media and materials Imagination Responding to experiences, and expressing and communicating ideas	120 124 126

Ideas for organising the activity

This activity can be carried out using scraps of fabric from clothes that children have worn out. This provides an opportunity for children to talk about where they wore the clothes and why they liked them. It works well with individual children or pairs, as most children will need adult support and supervision while using fabric scissors.

Begin by reading the Elmer story and talk about friendship. Check that children understand the concept of something being a patchwork.

Ask children if they can cut out squares from the fabric that they have chosen. Encourage them to talk about the fabric that they are using. Once they have cut out squares or rectangles, ask them to choose a place on the card to stick them onto. Would they like to decorate the squares further, e.g. sticking on beads, sequins or lace? The finished board can be displayed with a frame or border.

Extending and varying children's learning

◆ Children can make their own patchwork.
◆ Children can sew items such as buttons onto their patchwork.
◆ Show children real patchwork quilts and eiderdowns.

Theme 8 Homes

'Homes' is a good starting point and, if children become interested, it can be extended to look at homes of animals, buildings and things in the home.

Inside the box on each area of learning below is a range of ideas for activities and stories on the theme of homes. You will find on the following pages a ready-made activity plan for the first idea listed in each box. In addition, all the stories mentioned are listed in the Booklist on pages 250–252.

Ideas to suggest to parents
◆ Point out house numbers and street names.
◆ Point out different types of homes, e.g. flats, semi-detached, terraced.
◆ Show their child chimneys and other features of homes such as windows.

Personal, social and emotional development
◆ *Activity plan: Jobs around the home (p. 120)*
◆ Bring in a photo of you at home.
◆ What is your routine at home?
◆ Keeping safe at home – objects that are safe and unsafe.
◆ Do you have a favourite place at home?
◆ Guess where teddy's favourite place is?

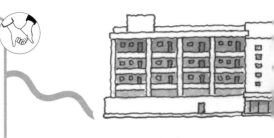

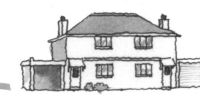

Communication, language and literacy
◆ *Activity plan: Can this go in the home? (p. 121)*
◆ Kim's game: Things that are found in many homes.
◆ Picture lotto: Things that go in homes.
◆ Role-play area: In the bedroom.
◆ Which items are in the kitchen?
◆ Rhyme: 'The old woman who lived in the shoe'
◆ Stories:
  ◆ *The Do-It-Yourself House that Jack Built*
  ◆ *In My Bathroom*
  ◆ *Kipper*
  ◆ *Kitten Finds a Home*
  ◆ *Percy the Park Keeper and the Storm*
  ◆ *Teddy Bears Moving Day*

Creative development

- *Activity plan: Make your own den (p. 126)*
- Display: Street scene – houses, shops, trees with birds' nests.
- Can you paint a picture of where you live?
- Look at this wallpaper – can you make your own prints?
- Role play: Estate agents.
- Make a picture for your room.
- Small world play – doll's house.
- Camping – with these sheets can you make your own tent?

Physical development

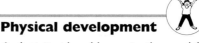

- *Activity plan: Homes in the sand (p. 125)*
- Let's pretend we are moving house – can you pack these boxes?
- Three little pigs – can you make a home out of these materials?
- Can you find the missing key hidden outdoors?
- Can you turn the key in the lock – which lock fits which key?
- Tents and tunnels in the outdoor play area.

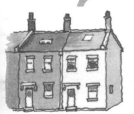

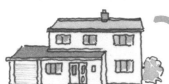

Knowledge and understanding of the world

- *Activity plan: Things we do at home (p. 123)*
- Can you see any homes belonging to spiders, birds or other creatures?
- Make a home for this teddy.
- Look at these photos – are these homes new or old?
- Doors – what types of doors do homes have?
- Dice game – the house that Jack built.
- Bird's nest or wasp's nest for children to observe.
- Walk around the area – what homes can we see?
- Make a map to show your journey here – what do you see?

Mathematical development

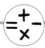

- *Activity plan: Which home is the best fit? (p. 122)*
- Ordering keys – size, shape.
- Doll's house furniture to sort – things that go in homes.
- Doors – what number do you live at?
- Teddy's forgotten which wallpaper he used. Can you help him to match this piece?
- How many keys can you feel in this bag – one, two, three or more?
- Let's look at the buildings around us – what shapes can we see?
- Game – the house that Jack built.

Activity plans for the theme 'homes'

I Jobs around the home

Hello teddy – what have you been doing? You have been doing some jobs in the home. I wonder if the children would like to have a go at some of the jobs that you have been doing?

Specific resources

- teddy or other stooge
- items to be washed up
- cloths
- washing-up bowl
- aprons
- tea towels

Key learning intentions

This activity is designed to help children's sense of community and to develop their physical skills.

Links to Foundation Stage curriculum

Area of learning	Aspects of learning	Curriculum guidance page
Personal, social and emotional development	Disposition and attitudes Self-confidence and self-esteem Making relationships Self-care Sense of community	32 34 36 40 42
Communication, language and literacy	Language for communication Language for thinking Handwriting	48, 50, 52, 54 56–8 66
Knowledge and understanding of the world	Exploration and investigation Sense of time Cultures and beliefs	86, 88 94 98
Physical development	Movement Using equipment Using tools and materials	106, 108 112 114
Creative development	Imagination	124

Ideas for organising the activity

This activity works well with small groups of children or pairs. Decide beforehand on some tasks the children can do, such as washing up, polishing shoes, wiping tables, sorting out toys.

Using teddy as a stooge: ask the children to guess what he has been doing to help. Ask them why it is important to help out around the home and the setting. What tasks has teddy been doing? Have they ever helped out at home? What do they know how to do?

Ask the children if they would like to show teddy the things that they can do to help. Move teddy with you while they are helping and carry on a conversation with him, e.g. 'Look how Wayne is able to tidy up!' This type of activity is important as it boosts children's self-esteem whilst developing the all-important fine motor skills that will be needed later in writing.

Health and safety
This type of activity needs to be closely supervised. It is important to know if any children have skin conditions that might mean they should not have contact with washing-up liquid.

Extending and varying children's learning
- Take photographs of the children at work – encourage parents to give children some responsibility at home.
- Sort out different cloths according to their uses.
- Ask the children to report back to teddy's mother on his day with them.
- Develop cleaning as a theme and provide things for the home corner.
- Put out magazines selling cleaning products, machines and gadgets – do the children recognise what they are and how they are used?

2 Can this go in the home?

Look at all these objects. Can we sort them out? Which ones would you put in a home? Why?

Specific resources
- items associated with the home, e.g. bedding, curtains, saucepans
- items not usually associated with the home, e.g. office equipment, spanner

Key learning intentions
This activity is designed to help children use language for thought and extend their vocabulary.

Links to Foundation Stage curriculum		
Area of learning	**Aspects of learning**	**Curriculum guidance page**
Personal, social and emotional development	Disposition and attitudes Behaviour and self-control Sense of community	32 38 42
Communication, language and literacy	Language for communication Language for thinking	48, 50, 52, 54 56–8
Mathematical development	Numbers as labels and for counting Shape, space and measures	74 78–80
Knowledge and understanding of the world	Exploration and investigation Sense of time Sense of place Cultures and beliefs	86, 88 94 96 98
Physical development	Using tools and materials	114
Creative development	Exploring media and materials	120

Ideas for organising the activity

This activity works best with small groups of children. Put several objects out for children to touch and explore. Ask them if they can name the objects – what are they used for? Explain to them the purpose of any unusual objects they may not have recognised.

Using a stooge ask the children to choose one object at a time and tell the stooge where it belongs. The stooge can ask the child questions to clarify further. Can the children count the number of objects? Which objects are the odd ones out? Which objects can be found both in the home and outside the home?

Use this activity as a way of encouraging children to talk about items that they have at home.

Extending and varying children's learning

◆ Children can draw some of the objects.
◆ Stooge can ask the children to write them a note so that he can remember everything.
◆ Which rooms do these objects belong in?
◆ Put smaller objects in a feely bag – can the children recognise them?

3 Which home is the best fit?

Look at these homes made from Lego. Which home would be the best fit for this cuddly toy?

Specific resources

◆ Lego or Duplo bricks, small cuddly toy or plastic animal

> **Key learning intentions**
> This activity is designed to help children consider size and shape and to use positional language.

Links to Foundation Stage curriculum		
Area of learning	**Aspects of learning**	**Curriculum guidance page**
Personal, social and emotional development	Disposition and attitudes Making relationships Behaviour and self-control Self-care Sense of community	32 36 38 40 42
Communication, language and literacy	Language for communication Language for thinking Writing	48, 50, 52, 54 56–8 64
Mathematical development	Numbers as labels and for counting Calculating Shape, space and measures	74 76 78–80
Knowledge and understanding of the world	Exploration and investigation Designing and making skills	86, 88 90

▽

| Physical development | Movement
Using tools and materials | 106, 108
114 |
| Creative development | Exploring media and materials
Imagination | 120
124 |

Ideas for organising the activity

This activity works well with individuals or pairs. Begin by building three houses of different sizes from Lego or Duplo bricks – two of which should be too small for the cuddly toy or animal to fit inside.

Show the children the cuddly toy or plastic animal and let them play with it if necessary. Can they decide which would be the best house? Encourage them to try the different houses. Which house is the largest? Which house do they think is the nicest?

Use this activity as a way of encouraging children to talk about their homes and what they like about their homes. Once they have played with this activity, encourage them to go and build a home to fit the animal. They can also write a note to tell the animal that the house is ready!

Extending and varying children's learning

◆ Ask children to take one of the smaller houses – can they make it large enough?
◆ Ask children if they can make a house out of only a certain number of bricks.
◆ Ask children to make a house that has three storeys.

4 Things we do at home

Look at all these photographs. Which of these things do you do at home? Do you sleep, clean your teeth, watch television?

Specific resources

◆ magazines about homes   ◆ paper   ◆ crayons
◆ paints   ◆ pencils   ◆ other materials available for display
◆ photographs of children playing with toys or doing things at home

> **Key learning intentions**
> This activity is to help children to think about things that most people do at home. It should help children become aware of the differences and similarities between them.

Links to Foundation Stage curriculum		
Area of learning	**Aspects of learning**	**Curriculum guidance page**
Personal, social and emotional development	Disposition and attitudes Self-confidence and self-esteem Making relationships Behaviour and self-control Sense of community	32 34 36 38 42

▽

Communication, language and literacy	Language for communication Language for thinking Linking sounds with letters Reading Writing Handwriting	48, 50, 52, 54 56–8 60 62 64 66
Mathematical development	Shape, space and measures	78–80
Knowledge and understanding of the world	Designing and making skills Sense of time Sense of place Cultures and beliefs	90 94 96 98
Physical development	Movement Using tools and materials	106, 108 114
Creative development	Exploring media and materials Responding to experiences, and expressing and communicating ideas	120 126

Ideas for organising the activity

This activity works well with small groups of children or pairs. The aim should be to allow children to talk about themselves and their homes freely. Begin by putting out a selection of photographs and magazines for children to look at. Ask them to find photos of things that they do at home. Ask children to think about what they do in

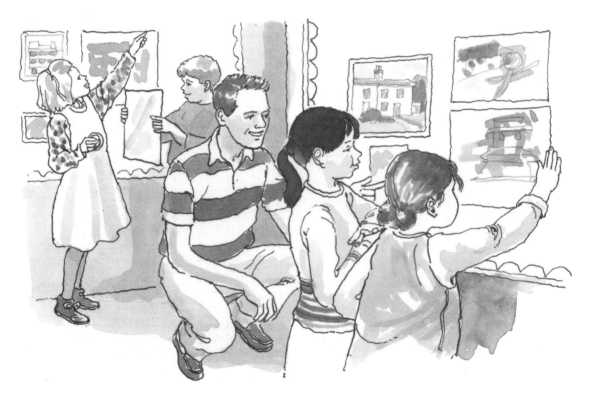

Encourage children to put the display together as this will help their sense of measuring and space

the morning, e.g. wash, have breakfast, clean teeth, get dressed, etc. Can they find pictures that show children doing these things or the places where they happen, e.g. bathroom, kitchen?

Check that they know the words for rooms of the house and items within them. This is especially important for children who have more than one language as they may only hear these nouns in their home language, which may not be English.

Put out pencils, crayons and other drawing materials. Can children do a drawing of some of the things they like doing at home? Use the drawings and photos that they have made or cut out to form the basis of the display. Encourage children to help put the display together as this will help their sense of measuring and space.

Extending and varying children's learning

◆ Children can 'write' about their pictures.
◆ Encourage children to notice the shape of the 'h' in home and house.
◆ Use sequencing cards for children to work out what they do first, second and third in the morning.
◆ Children can cut out pictures of their favourite toys and stick these onto a picture of a sitting room or a bedroom.

5 Homes in the sand

Look at this dinosaur. Can you make a home for it in the sand tray?

Specific resources

◆ scoops   ◆ small containers   ◆ sand, either in a sand pit or in small trays
◆ plastic animals such as farm animals or dinosaurs
◆ hand-held vacuum cleaner for children to hoover up sand after activity

---

Key learning intentions
This activity should help children's fine manipulative skills and hand-eye co-ordination whilst encouraging role play.

Links to Foundation Stage curriculum		
Area of learning	**Aspects of learning**	**Curriculum guidance page**
Personal, social and emotional development	Disposition and attitudes Behaviour and self-control Self-care Sense of community	32 38 40 42
Communication, language and literacy	Language for communication Language for thinking Handwriting	48, 50, 52, 54 56–8 66

▽

Mathematical development	Shape, space and measures	78–80
Knowledge and understanding of the world	Exploration and investigation Designing and making skills Information and communication technology	86, 88 90 92
Physical development	Movement Using tools and materials	106, 108 114
Creative development	Exploring media and materials Imagination Responding to experiences, and expressing and communicating ideas	120 124 126

Ideas for organising the activity

This activity can be carried out in a large sand pit, or sand can be put into smaller trays so that children can play individually with the sand. Show the children the animal and ask them if they could make it a home – perhaps a cave, a tunnel or a castle. Encourage them to experiment with different ways of making the animal a home. How big will it need to be? Will the animal need a series of rooms or places to play?

Use this activity as a way of helping children to talk about their own homes as well as a way of modelling positional language. Once children have finished playing with the sand, encourage them to hoover up any sand that has fallen on the floor with the hand-held vacuum cleaner. This will help them to use ICT.

Extending and varying children's learning

- Encourage the children to make items for the animal's home, e.g. somewhere to lie down, a garden path, etc.
- Children can build a sand neighbourhood for several animals to live in.
- Ask children about the rules of the 'house' – is there anything that the animal should or should not do to keep his home nice?

6 Make your own den

Look at these large boxes and sheets that we have here today. Can you make yourselves a den or somewhere to hide?

Specific resources

- large cardboard boxes
- tablecloths
- sheets
- pieces of fabric

Key learning intentions
This activity will help children to explore materials creatively. It will also encourage spatial awareness.

Links to Foundation Stage curriculum		
Area of learning	**Aspects of learning**	**Curriculum guidance page**
Personal, social and emotional development	Disposition and attitudes Self-confidence and self-esteem Making relationships Behaviour and self-control Self-care Sense of community	32 34 36 38 40 42
Communication, language and literacy	Language for communication Language for thinking	48, 50, 52, 54 56–8
Mathematical development	Shape, space and measures	78–80
Knowledge and understanding of the world	Exploration and investigation Designing and making skills Sense of place Cultures and beliefs	86, 88 90 96 98
Physical development	Sense of space Movement Health and bodily awareness Using equipment Using tools and materials	104 106, 108 110 112 114
Creative development	Exploring media and materials Imagination Responding to experiences, and expressing and communicating ideas	120 124 126

Ideas for organising the activity

This activity needs to be placed where children will be able to build and stay in their dens. Younger children will need an adult to help them build, while reception-age children should be able to build a den/tent in pairs or very small groups. Begin by showing them the materials available.

Ask the children to think of things they need to consider when building a den, e.g. it has to be big enough for them to get inside. Encourage them to build their dens, supporting and helping them where needed. Encourage them to collect things that they can put inside their den.

Use this as an opportunity for children to work together and also to talk about homes.

Extending and varying children's learning

◆ Encourage children to make things such as tables out of smaller boxes for their den.
◆ Provide children with props for their dens such as tea sets, games.
◆ Take photographs of the process of building the den.
◆ Ask children if they can visit each other's den.
◆ Ask children if they can build a den for the staff!
◆ Provide different materials for children to use, e.g. boxes, blankets.
◆ Encourage children to make their own snacks to eat in their den.
◆ Read *Mr Bear's Holiday*.

Theme 9 Hospitals

This theme, based on the story *I Don't Want to go to Hospital* by Tony Ross (Picture Lions), is interesting because some children will have visited or been in hospital, while many will have visited doctors or dentists. Within the story of the princess who did not want to go to hospital there is also the theme of hiding and being afraid.

Inside the box on each area of learning below is a range of ideas for activities and stories on the theme of hospitals. You will find on the following pages a ready-made activity plan for the first idea listed in each box. In addition, all the stories mentioned are listed in the Booklist on pages 250–252.

Ideas to suggest to parents
- ◆ Point out ambulances when they are out and about.
- ◆ Show their child where their doctor and dental practices are.
- ◆ Talk to their child about not touching medicines or tablets.

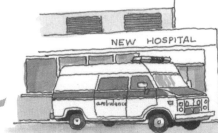

Personal, social and emotional development
- ◆ *Activity plan: I don't like it when … (p. 130)*
- ◆ Show teddy how you clean your teeth.
- ◆ Hand washing – which of these soaps do you like best?
- ◆ Poor teddy is feeling poorly – how can you make him feel better?
- ◆ Were you born in a hospital – have you any photographs or name bands?

Communication, language and literacy
- ◆ *Activity plan: Sequence the story (p. 131)*
- ◆ Stories:
  - ◆ *Freddie Visits the Doctor*
  - ◆ *I Don't Want to go to Hospital*
  - ◆ *Owl at the Vet*
  - ◆ *Topsy and Tim go to Hospital*
  - ◆ *Topsy and Tim go to the Dentist*
- ◆ Role play: Animal hospital, at the opticians
- ◆ Songs:
  - ◆ 'Head, shoulders, knees and toes'
  - ◆ 'Simon says'
- ◆ Writing area – clipboards, paper and pens.

Creative development

- *Activity plan: Role-play area: Hospitals (p. 136)*
- When the music stops pretend to be asleep so that the tooth fairy can come by.
- What sounds can your body make?
- Songs:
  - 'Head, shoulders, knees and toes'
  - 'I have got a body' (*Game Songs with Prof Dog's Troupe*)
  - 'One finger, one thumb keep moving …'

Physical development

- *Activity plan: Princess hide and seek (p. 135)*
- Tricycles and large equipment – transport the dolls and cuddly toys to hospital.
- Visitor: A dentist – how can we look after our teeth?
- Can you run really quickly – how does your body feel?
- Can you listen to each other's heartbeat?
- Bite into an apple – can you see your teeth marks?

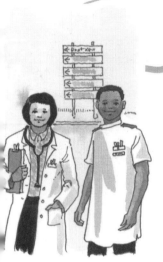

Knowledge and understanding of the world

- *Activity plan: Get-well cards (p. 133)*
- Have you ever been ill or felt poorly?
- Where is the dentist or doctor in your area?
- X-rays and scans – look at these pictures.
- Can you sort these glasses – which ones are sunglasses?
- Visit by a health worker, e.g. doctor.

Mathematical development

- *Activity plan: Which bandage is the longest? (p. 132)*
- Which will hold more water – a medicine spoon or a tablespoon?
- How many medicine spoonfuls of water fill a small bottle?
- Roll a dice – put spoonfuls of sand into a bottle according to the number on the dice – first to fill the bottle wins.
- How many teeth have you got – can you count them?

Activity plans for the theme 'hospitals'

1 I don't like it when . . .

This book is about a little girl who felt afraid. It is a lovely story because in the end she becomes very happy.

Specific resources

◆ *I Don't Want to go to Hospital* by Tony Ross
◆ other books about feeling nervous or afraid
◆ collage materials
◆ paints
◆ paper and crayons

Key learning intentions
This activity should help children to acknowledge their feelings of being frightened or unhappy.

Links to Foundation Stage curriculum

Area of learning	Aspects of learning	Curriculum guidance page
Personal, social and emotional development	Disposition and attitudes Self-confidence and self-esteem Making relationships Behaviour and self-control Sense of community	32 34 36 38 42
Communication, language and literacy	Language for communication Language for thinking Handwriting	48, 50, 52, 54 56–8 66
Knowledge and understanding of the world	Sense of time Sense of place Cultures and beliefs	94 96 98
Physical development	Sense of space Movement Using tools and materials	104 106, 108 114
Creative development	Exploring media and materials Imagination Responding to experiences, and expressing and communicating ideas	120 124 126

Ideas for organising the activity

This activity should be done with pairs or small groups of children, so that they can speak freely. Read the story *I Don't Want to go to Hospital* with the children. Ask them if they can understand why the princess did not want to go to hospital. Ask them if they have ever felt frightened or not wanted to go somewhere. What things make them feel scared – dogs, night-time, loud noises, etc.? Show them the paper, paint and materials and ask them to show how they feel when they are scared or unhappy. Encourage them to think about things that make them feel better, e.g. a hug from a parent, a smile from a friend.

With the children put up a display of their drawings and representations. Encourage them to 'write' about their work.

Extending and varying children's learning

◆ Ask children if they would like to make a get-well card for the princess.
◆ Produce a display about things that make children happy.
◆ Put teddy in a bag with a torch and make up a story about teddy being afraid of the night.
◆ Read stories such as *The Owl Who Was Afraid of the Dark*.

2 Sequence the story

Here are five pictures from the story *I Don't Want to go to Hospital*. Can you work out the order they should be in?

Specific resources

◆ photocopies of five of the illustrations from *I Don't Want to go to Hospital*
◆ pencils   ◆ crayons

> **Key learning intentions**
> This activity is designed to help children sequence and retell the story.

Links to Foundation Stage curriculum		
Area of learning	**Aspects of learning**	**Curriculum guidance page**
Personal, social and emotional development	Disposition and attitudes	32
Communication, language and literacy	Language for communication Language for thinking Linking sounds with letters Reading Writing	48, 50, 52, 54 56–8 60 62 64
Mathematical development	Shape, space and measures	78–80
Knowledge and understanding of the world	Sense of time	94
Physical development	Using tools and materials	114
Creative development	Responding to experiences, and expressing and communicating ideas	126

Ideas for organising the activity

This activity works well with pairs of children or individuals. Read the story *I Don't Want to go to Hospital* or ask the children to retell it if it has recently been read.

Show the children the photocopied pages. Can they remember what was happening? Can they put the pages in the correct order? Help them if needed by bringing out the book so that they can match the pictures to the story.

Ask the children to 'write' the story of what is happening in their 'own' words onto one of the sheets.

Extending and varying children's learning

◆ Children can paint a picture of one of the characters in the story.
◆ Encourage children to act out the story using props.

3 Which bandage is the longest?

Have a look at these bandages. How many are there? Which one do you think is the longest? Now unroll them. Were you right?

Specific resources

◆ crepe bandages of three different lengths (or more depending on the children)

Key learning intentions
This activity will help children to measure and use mathematical language such as 'longest', 'shortest'. It will also help them to count.

Links to Foundation Stage curriculum		
Area of learning	**Aspects of learning**	**Curriculum guidance page**
Personal, social and emotional development	Disposition and attitudes	32
Communication, language and literacy	Language for communication Language for thinking Reading Writing	48, 50, 52, 54 56–8 62 64
Mathematical development	Numbers as labels and for counting Calculating Shape, space and measures	74 76 78–80
Knowledge and understanding of the world	Exploration and investigation	86, 88
Physical development	Using tools and materials	114
Creative development	Exploring media and materials	120

Ideas for organising the activity

This activity works well with pairs or small groups of children. Put out the bandages, and let them play with them if they have not had an opportunity to touch and feel bandages before. How do they feel? Are they soft? Roll up the bandages and ask the children if they can count how many there are. Ask them to predict which one will be the longest. Let the children unroll them and then compare them.

Model language for them and encourage them to talk about why they have decided that one is longer than another. Write labels for two of the bandages –

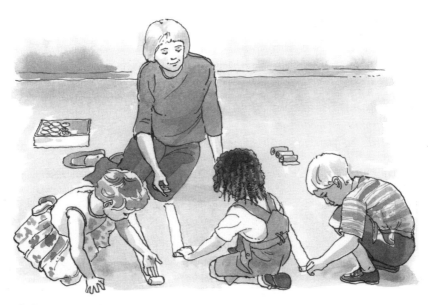

Encourage them to talk about why they have decided that one is longer than another

'longest', 'shortest', so that children can see an adult writing. Can the children put the labels next to the right bandages? The children can also 'write' their own labels to help them remember.

Ask the children if they can roll up the bandages (some children will find this very difficult!).

Health and safety
Make sure the bandages are not left unsupervised in case children decide to put them around their necks.

Extending and varying children's learning
- Using cuddly toys such as teddies and dolls, ask children to choose the best bandage for one part of its body, e.g. teddy's arm.
- Produce a display showing shortest and longest.
- See if children can find objects in the room that are the same length as one of the bandages.

4 Get-well cards
Let's make some get-well cards for the role-play area. Here are some get-well cards that people send.

Specific resources
- get-well cards
- paper
- felt tips
- collage materials
- children's name cards
- card
- crayons
- scissors
- letters of the alphabet
- paints
- ribbons
- other materials children will enjoy touching and using

Key learning intentions

This activity will encourage children to choose materials and use them independently. It will also encourage them to 'write'.

Links to Foundation Stage curriculum

Area of learning	Aspects of learning	Curriculum guidance page
Personal, social and emotional development	Disposition and attitudes Self-confidence and self-esteem Self-care	32 34 40
Communication, language and literacy	Language for communication Language for thinking Linking sounds with letters Reading Writing	48, 50, 52, 54 56–8 60 62 64
Mathematical development	Shape, space and measures	78–80
Knowledge and understanding of the world	Exploration and investigation Designing and making skills Information and communication technology	86, 88 90 92
Physical development	Using equipment Using tools and materials	112 114
Creative development	Exploring media and materials Imagination Responding to experiences, and expressing and communicating ideas	120 124 126

Ideas for organising the activity

Begin with the story *I Don't Want to go to Hospital*. Ask the children if they remember what the doctor said the princess would get in hospital (sweets and cards). Show children examples of get-well cards. (If they are interested in reading and letters, point out the 'get' 'well' words to them.)

Ask the children if they would like to make get-well cards for the role-play area. Show them the different materials. For the children to be creative in this activity, it will be important for them to be supported rather than directed.

Once they have finished making their cards, encourage them to write a message inside and sign their names. Provide name cards and letters so that they can remember the shapes of letters. The final cards can be used in the role-play area or put on display.

Extending and varying children's learning

◆ Encourage children to make other items for the role-play area such as notices, menus, posters and pictures.
◆ Provide a selection of cards and see if children can sort out birthday cards from get-well cards.
◆ Make get-well cards to send to the local hospital.
◆ Make envelopes for the cards to go in.

5 Princess hide and seek

Do you remember that, in the story, the princess tries to hide and everyone looks for her? Can you see where the princess is hiding? The other children know. When they make very loud sounds, you will know you are getting closer.

Specific resources

- musical instruments such as shakers
- rattles
- a doll or puppet to be the princess

Key learning intentions

This activity is designed to develop children's auditory discrimination and their spatial awareness.

Links to Foundation Stage curriculum		
Area of learning	**Aspects of learning**	**Curriculum guidance page**
Personal, social and emotional development	Disposition and attitudes Behaviour and self-control	32 38
Communication, language and literacy	Language for communication Linking sounds with letters	48, 50, 52, 54 60
Mathematical development	Shape, space and measures	78–80
Physical development	Sense of space Movement	104 106, 108
Creative development	Music	122

Ideas for organising the activity

This activity works well with groups of children. Begin by letting them choose a musical instrument. If they have not used instruments for a while, encourage them to explore the sounds they make. Once they have finished 'exploring' tell them that they are going to play a game. Practise with children making loud and then soft sounds.

Show them the doll or puppet that is to be hidden. Ask one child to close their eyes or step away from the main group while another child hides it. When the child comes back the other children must make plenty of sound if the child is getting close to it, but be very quiet if the child is moving away from it.

Extending and varying children's learning

- Children can play the game in pairs – one child hides an object, the other has to find it.
- Children can play name treasure hunts (see p. 165).
- Play hide and seek with pairs – but the child who is looking for the object must ask questions to work out where it is hidden.
- Ask the children to paint or draw a picture and hide the princess somewhere in it.

6 Role-play area: Hospitals

Do you want to play in the hospital? Who is feeling ill? Who is looking after the patient? What will the patient need?

Specific resources

- beds
- pretend first-aid kits
- computer keyboards
- bandages
- crutches
- uniforms
- pencils and charts
- washing-up bowls
- magazines for a waiting area
- play stethoscopes
- telephones
- towels
- wheelchairs

(Ask your local hospital, health visitor or health promotion unit if they have anything that can be borrowed.)

Key learning intentions
The aim of this activity is to extend children's vocabulary and to play co-operatively.

Links to Foundation Stage curriculum		
Area of learning	**Aspects of learning**	**Curriculum guidance page**
Personal, social and emotional development	Disposition and attitudes Self-confidence and self-esteem Making relationships Behaviour and self-control Self-care	32 34 36 38 40
Communication, language and literacy	Language for communication Language for thinking Reading Writing Handwriting	48, 50, 52, 54 56–8 62 64 66
Mathematical development	Numbers as labels and for counting	74
Knowledge and understanding of the world	Exploration and investigation	86, 88
Physical development	Sense of space Health and bodily awareness Using equipment Using tools and materials	104 110 112 114
Creative development	Imagination Responding to experiences, and expressing and communicating ideas	124 126

Ideas for organising the activity

For successful role play in this area, children will need to have some input first. Read stories about hospitals, use visitors, or role play what might happen in a hospital. Show children what specific pieces of equipment are used for, e.g. stethoscope to listen to the heartbeat, thermometer to feel their temperature. Make sure children learn that doctors and nurses write things down so that children can role play writing on charts, books – both numbers and letters. Children may remember what it is like to feel ill – and what cheers them up, e.g. toys, having drinks poured for them. Use the washing-up bowl with a little water so that children can wash their hands before touching patients or pretend to wash dolls faces.

To avoid sex stereotyping, make sure children see images of male and female nurses and doctors and intervene if necessary if play appears sex-typed.

Extending and varying children's learning

◆ Making items for the role-play area, e.g. trolleys, drinks and foods for the patients.
◆ Encourage children to find items that will cheer up the patients.

Theme 10 Me

This is a traditional yet effective starting point, especially useful when children first come into settings. It lends itself to children talking about their homes and important events in their lives – all important when getting to know children.

Inside the box on each area of learning below is a range of ideas for activities and stories on the theme of me. You will find on the following pages a ready-made activity plan for the first idea listed in each box. In addition, all the stories mentioned are listed in the Booklist on pages 250–252.

Ideas to suggest to parents
◆ Compare hand sizes with their child.
◆ Encourage their child to look in the mirror – what colour eyes have they got?
◆ Show pictures of their child when they were younger – what can they remember?
◆ Talk to their child about things that they used to when they were children.

Personal, social and emotional development

◆ *Activity plan: My special things (p. 140)*
◆ Ways in which I can help.
◆ Stories:
  ◆ *Can't You Sleep, Little Bear?*
  ◆ *Helpers*
  ◆ *My Mum and Dad Make Me Laugh*
◆ Draw a picture of the people you live with.
◆ Things I can do for myself.
◆ Teddy needs a friend – how can he be a good friend?
◆ I like it when ... I don't like it when ...

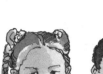

Communication, language and literacy

◆ *Activity plan: Let's guess what is in your hands (p. 141)*
◆ Stories:
  ◆ *Big Book of Families*
  ◆ *Hello Toes! Hello Feet!*
  ◆ *I Like It When*
  ◆ *Mum and Me*
  ◆ *My Own Big Bed*
  ◆ *Wash, Scrub, Brush*
  ◆ *Would You Rather*
  ◆ *You Smell*
◆ Hunt your name in the room.
◆ Can you post your name in the box?
◆ Role-play area: In my bedroom.
◆ Display: My favourite foods.

Creative development

- *Activity plan: Musical follow my leader (p. 146)*
- Mix paint with your hands.
- Make patterns and marks with your fist, palms, fingers.
- Resources for movement such as music tapes.
- *Shake, Rattle, Roll.*
- Look in the mirror – what can you see? – how many faces can you make?
- Draw self – draw each other.
- Who is hiding – can you recognise their voice?
- Favourite songs – which ones do you like best?

Physical development

- *Activity plan: Giant steps, tiny steps (p. 145)*
- How many ways can you find to move around the outdoor area?
- Can you get from this side to the other without stepping on the floor?
- How far/high can you throw this beanbag?
- Against the egg timer – how many jumps can you make?
- Can you tip toe along a chalk line?
- Can you take a friend around an obstacle course?
- Can you hop or jump into these squares?

Knowledge and understanding of the world

- *Activity plan: A book about me (p. 144)*
- Do you know your address and phone number?
- Make a phone call home.
- Who is the oldest/youngest person in your family?
- What is your favourite place in this area – park, swimming pool, shops?
- My special days – bring in photos.
- Walk – what can we see today?
- Smells – which of these smells sweet, sour, strong?
- Touch – find the softest, hardest, furriest item.
- Sing into the tape recorder – your favourite song.

Mathematical development

- *Activity plan: How much can my hand hold? (p. 143)*
- How many people are in your family?
- Draw around your shoes – who has the biggest shoes?
- How old am I? Put the candles into the cake (dough).
- How old is teddy today? Count the candles.
- How heavy are you?
- Things that are smaller than me.

Activity plans for the theme 'me'

I My special things

Have you got a photograph of or can you draw some things that are special for you?
Perhaps you may be able to bring some things in.

Specific resources

- materials for a wall or table display
- materials to help children draw or catalogues for children to cut out pictures
- items brought in from home

> **Key learning intentions**
> This activity is designed to help children feel valued and to talk about things that are
> important in their lives, such as toys, clothes, photographs, etc.

Links to Foundation Stage curriculum

Area of learning	Aspects of learning	Curriculum guidance page
Personal, social and emotional development	Disposition and attitudes Self-confidence and self-esteem Making relationships Behaviour and self-control Self-care Sense of community	32 34 36 38 40 42
Communication, language and literacy	Language for communication Language for thinking Reading Writing	48, 50, 52, 54 56–8 62 64
Mathematical development	Shape, space and measures	78–80
Knowledge and understanding of the world	Exploration and investigation Sense of time Cultures and beliefs	86, 88 94 98
Physical development	Movement Using tools and materials	106, 108 114
Creative development	Exploring media and materials Responding to experiences, and expressing and communicating ideas	120 126

Ideas for organising the activity

This activity should be carried out with individual children or pairs, as it should
encourage children to talk about what they have brought in or are trying to
draw / write about. The role of the adult here is to listen!

Children should also be involved with making the display – there may be some
challenges as to how best to display things. This activity should also be a good
opportunity to talk about respecting people's special things. If items are very special,
children could be encouraged to draw, paint or record them.

Extending and varying children's learning

◆ Make up stories about favourite things that get lost, e.g. teddy has lost his favourite sock.
◆ Encourage children to ask each other about the items that have been brought in.
◆ Ask children if they can find their name cards to put next to their item or representation.
◆ Count the number of items that are similar, e.g. how many clothes, toys, etc.

2 Let's guess what is in your hands

Choose an object. Put it in your hands. Can we all guess what you have in your hands?

Specific resources

◆ small objects that can be put in hands such as:
◆ small toys   ◆ keys   ◆ cottons

Key learning intentions
This activity is designed to promote children's overall language development, especially their ability to use language for thinking and describing.

Links to Foundation Stage curriculum		
Area of learning	**Aspects of learning**	**Curriculum guidance page**
Personal, social and emotional development	Disposition and attitudes Making relationships Behaviour and self-control Self-care Sense of community	32 36 38 40 42
Communication, language and literacy	Language for communication Language for thinking Linking sounds with letters	48, 50, 52, 54 56–8 60
Mathematical development	Shape, space and measures	78–80
Knowledge and understanding of the world	Exploration and investigation	86, 88

Ideas for organising the activity

Put out a selection of objects for children to look at and touch. Work with a small group of children, even pairs. Ask a child to choose an object and then enclose it in their hands.

You can either encourage children to ask questions about what the object is or you can ask the child to keep looking at the object and tell the others about it. Can they guess what it is?

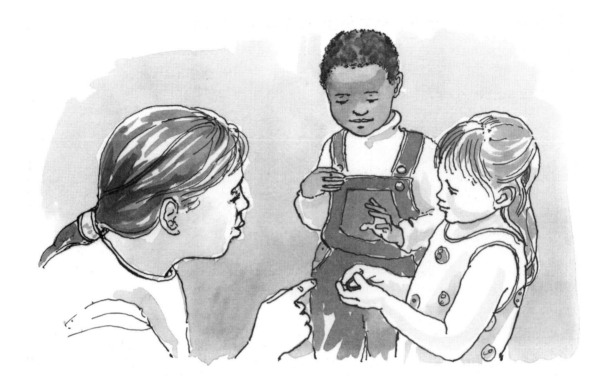

Can they guess what the object is?

Health and safety
Choose objects you feel will be suitable for children to handle and play with.

Extending and varying children's learning

◆ Count how many objects are on the tray.
◆ Children can make their own feely bags to play this game.
◆ Use a stooge such as a puppet to play the game so that children can hear the language modelled.
◆ Encourage the children to play this game in pairs so that they choose items together.

3 How much can my hand hold? $=^+_\times-$

Look at this sand. How much sand can you hold in your hand? Will it fill this beaker?

Specific resources
◆ beaker ◆ sand

Key learning intentions
This activity helps children measure, compare and also problem solve.

Links to Foundation Stage curriculum		
Area of learning	**Aspects of learning**	**Curriculum guidance page**
Personal, social and emotional development	Disposition and attitudes Self-confidence and self-esteem Behaviour and self-control	32 34 38
Communication, language and literacy	Language for communication Language for thinking	48, 50, 52, 54 56–8
Mathematical development	Numbers as labels and for counting Calculating Shape, space and measures	74 76 78–80
Knowledge and understanding of the world	Exploration and investigation	86, 88
Physical development	Using tools and materials	114
Creative development	Exploring media and materials	120

Ideas for organising the activity

Using sand as a starting point, ask children how much sand they think they can hold in their hand. Ask them to put the sand in their hands into a beaker or other container. Whose hand holds the most? Is there more than one way of holding sand, e.g. palm open rather than clenched fist?

This activity should also provide opportunities for children to use the language of calculating, e.g. 'fewer', 'most', 'least'. It is a good idea to encourage them to fill up a container with sand and count how many handfuls they need to incorporate numbers as labels into this activity. If children are enjoying this activity they could also roll a dice and put in the number of handfuls shown on the dice – the first to fill a container has won.

Extending and varying children's learning
◆ How many handfuls of sand will be needed to fill the beaker or small bucket?
◆ Use other objects and repeat, e.g. buttons, marbles, feathers, rice, pasta.
◆ Compare adult handfuls with children's handfuls.
◆ Does it make any difference if sand is wet or dry?
◆ Draw around hands – did the child with the largest hand have the biggest handfuls?

4 A book about me

Here are some photographs with you in. Is that your family? Is there a photograph with your friends? Look, here is one that we took of you last week. Let's make these into your own book.

Specific resources
◆ paper ◆ pencils ◆ crayons
◆ photographs that children have brought in/have been taken in the setting

---

Key learning intentions

This activity helps children to develop a strong and positive self-image. It will also encourage children to talk about themselves and build relationships with their key workers.

Links to Foundation Stage curriculum		
Area of learning	**Aspects of learning**	**Curriculum guidance page**
Personal, social and emotional development	Disposition and attitudes Self-confidence and self-esteem Making relationships Self-care Sense of community	32 34 36 40 42
Communication, language and literacy	Language for communication Language for thinking Reading Writing	48, 50, 52, 54 56–8 62 64
Knowledge and understanding of the world	Sense of time Sense of place Cultures and beliefs	94 96 98
Physical development	Using tools and materials	114
Creative development	Exploring media and materials Responding to experiences, and expressing and communicating ideas	120 126

Ideas for organising the activity

Ask the child if they would like to make their own special book. Look at the photographs together and encourage the child to talk about them. Can they remember who they were with? Do they know where the photograph was taken? Encourage the child to work out an order in which they would like to put them in a book. Ask them if they would like to do their own 'writing' in the book, or scribe for them. They can then decorate their books choosing materials that they enjoy using. This activity should generate plenty of language and help each child feel valued.

Extending and varying children's learning
◆ Make a book about your setting with children.
◆ Make a poster or photo-collage of friends and family.
◆ Take photographs of the child at varying points of a session – can they put them in order?

5 Giant steps, tiny steps 🏃

Listen to this music – can you move to it using different steps?

Specific resources

◆ music with a strong beat or percussion drum

Key learning intentions

This activity is designed to help children's awareness of their bodies whilst developing their spatial awareness.

Links to Foundation Stage curriculum

Area of learning	Aspects of learning	Curriculum guidance page
Personal, social and emotional development	Disposition and attitudes Behaviour and self-control	32 38
Communication, language and literacy	Language for thinking Handwriting	56–8 66
Mathematical development	Shape, space and measures	78–80
Knowledge and understanding of the world	Information and communication technology	92
Physical development	Sense of space Movement	104 106, 108
Creative development	Exploring media and materials	120

Ideas for organising the activity

Using music or a percussion instrument, ask children if they can move or dance to it. Once they have enjoyed moving in their own ways to the music, ask them if they can make giant steps or strides as well as tip-toe steps. How far can they stride? Ask children if they can make small arm movements and then large arm movements such as circles in the air or up and down lines.

This activity can be developed into a game with children being given a signal to start moving in different ways. If you choose to use a tape or CD encourage children to be in charge of making it work. This will help them learn about ICT.

Extending and varying children's learning

◆ Read a story about a giant, e.g. *The Selfish Giant*.
◆ Put out dressing-up props such as hats, shoes, to help children take on different roles.
◆ See if the children can think about ways of measuring who has the largest stride.
◆ Look at ways of walking quickly and also slowly – who can walk the slowest?
◆ Roll a dice – how many strides can you take?

6 Musical follow my leader

Take an instrument, follow the leader. Shake and move as they do!

Specific resources
◆ selection of percussion instruments – shakers, etc.

> **Key learning intentions**
> This activity is designed to help children explore musical sounds and also to enjoy co-operating with others.

Links to Foundation Stage curriculum

Area of learning	Aspects of learning	Curriculum guidance page
Personal, social and emotional development	Disposition and attitudes Making relationships Behaviour and self-control Self-care Sense of community	32 36 38 40 42
Communication, language and literacy	Linking sounds with letters Handwriting	60 66
Knowledge and understanding of the world	Exploration and investigation	86, 88
Physical development	Sense of space Movement Using tools and materials	104 106, 108 114
Creative development	Exploring media and materials Music	120 122

Ideas for organising the activity

Begin this activity by encouraging children to choose their instruments. Allow them to play and explore the sounds they make. Can they make loud sounds? Soft sounds?

Encourage them to move as they make sounds. Can they remember to stop when they hear a special sound from you? Choose a child to be a leader. Can they follow the movements and the sounds?

Extending and varying children's learning

◆ Play this type of games using ribbons or scarves.
◆ Encourage children to work out the type of movements and sounds that they will make before becoming a leader.
◆ Play 'Simon says' games with musical instruments, i.e. when 'Simon says' they do, but if he doesn't they shouldn't make any sound!

Theme 11 Letters

Children love receiving letters and cards. This theme is a good starting point as it encourages children's early reading and writing skills.

Inside the box on each area of learning below is a range of ideas for activities and stories on the theme of letters. You will find on the following pages a ready-made activity plan for the first idea listed in each box. In addition, all the stories mentioned are listed in the Booklist on pages 250–252.

Ideas to suggest to parents
- Write their child a letter or a note.
- Take their child to a post office.
- Point out letter boxes and post office vans.
- Encourage their child to write a letter or do a drawing and post it to us.
- Read *Postman Pat* books.

Personal, social and emotional development
- *Activity plan: Postcards from all around the world (p. 150)*
- Display: Greeting cards, thank-you cards, Christmas cards, New Year cards, birthday cards.
- Each child to be sent a letter or a postcard – 'You're special because …'
- Here's a board – pin up your notes to each other.
- Make a thank-you letter/drawing to people who help us.

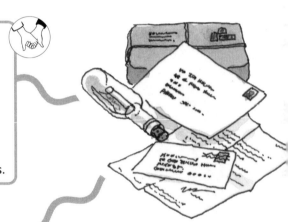

Communication, language and literacy
- *Activity plan: Message in a bottle (p. 151)*
- Emergent writing table – postcards, birthday cards, forms and envelopes.
- Finding and posting our names.
- Stories:
  - *Dear Zoo*
  - *King Rollo's Letter*
  - *A Letter to Granny*
  - *Postman Pat* series
- Role play: Card shop.
- Guess what might be in this envelope?
- Look at these envelopes teddy has brought – can you find yours?
- Write a letter to someone who is special to you.

Creative development

* *Activity plan: Making our own writing paper and envelopes (p. 156)*
* Role-play area: At the post office.
* Stamp and printing into dough.
* Make some tiny letters for the small world people.

Physical development

* *Activity plan: Delivering letters (p. 155)*
* Folding paper and putting it into envelopes.
* Envelopes in the sand tray – how many scoops to fill them?
* Teddy has hidden some letters outdoors for you to find.

Knowledge and understanding of the world

* *Activity plan: Sending e-mails and faxes (p. 153)*
* Where is the nearest post box to this setting? Can we post a letter there?
* Can you find two stamps the same?
* Sort stamps into piles: people/animals.
* Make your own post box.
* Visit your local post box or post office to send a letter.

Mathematical development

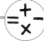

* *Activity plan: Forgetful teddy and his letters (p. 152)*
* How many letters have you got today?
* Which of these parcels is the heaviest?
* Put the number of stamps onto the envelopes – the boxes show you where to put the stamps.
* The card game – roll a dice and take the number of cards shown on the dice.
* Find the largest stamp, the smallest stamp.
* Count how many stamps are on this envelope.
* Find the right sized envelope for this piece of paper.

Activity plans for the theme 'letters'

1 Postcards from all around the world

Look at all the different postcards that we have received or have been brought in. Let's look at them and see if we recognise anywhere familiar.

Specific resources
◆ postcards showing local attractions
◆ postcards from people known to the children
◆ postcards brought from home

Key learning intentions
This activity is designed to help children to talk about their local environment as well as about being with their families on holidays.

Links to Foundation Stage curriculum		
Area of learning	**Aspects of learning**	**Curriculum guidance page**
Personal, social and emotional development	Disposition and attitudes Making relationships Behaviour and self-control Self-care	32 36 38 40
Communication, language and literacy	Language for communication Language for thinking Writing	48, 50, 52, 54 56–8 64
Mathematical development	Shape, space and measures	78–80
Knowledge and understanding of the world	Exploration and investigation Designing and making skills Sense of time	86, 88 90 94
Physical development	Using equipment Using tools and materials	112 114
Creative development	Exploring media and materials	120

Ideas for organising the activity
Before starting this theme, encourage people to send postcards into the setting. Collect postcards that show local attractions – contact the local tourist office.

Put about ten postcards at a time out for pairs or small groups of children to look at. Encourage them to take their time – looking at the pictures on the front as well as the stamps on the back. Can they remember going to any of these places? Do they think that the picture is taken in summer or winter? Which is their favourite postcard?

Extending and varying children's learning
◆ Play a game using three or four very different postcards. One child picks one up and describes what the picture is. All the cards are put out. Another child has to guess which postcard the child was describing.

◆ Sort the postcards out according to the scene, e.g. sea, buildings, bridges.
◆ Children write their own postcards to send.
◆ Children sort postcards with their favourite stamps into one pile.

2 Message in a bottle

Look, there's a bottle floating in the water tray. There seems to be a message inside. Shall we open it?

Specific resources

◆ small plastic bottles with lids
◆ crayons
◆ access to water tray
◆ letters and numbers to help children remember the shape of letters and numbers

◆ strips of paper
◆ pencils
◆ name cards

Key learning intentions
This activity will motivate children to write whilst finding out about objects that float.

Links to Foundation Stage curriculum		
Area of learning	**Aspects of learning**	**Curriculum guidance page**
Personal, social and emotional development	Disposition and attitudes Self-care	32 40
Communication, language and literacy	Language for communication Language for thinking Writing Handwriting	48, 50, 52, 54 56–8 64 66
Knowledge and understanding of the world	Exploration and investigation	86, 88
Physical development	Using equipment Using tools and materials	112 114
Creative development	Exploring media and materials	120

Ideas for organising the activity

Begin by putting a message from teddy or your stooge into a bottle and letting it float in the water tray. Ask the children what they think is in the bottle. How exciting! Tell them that sometimes people have written messages in bottles for other people to find. Open the bottle and read the message.

Ask the children if they would like to write their own messages. Who would they write a message to? Put out bottles, strips of paper, crayons and pencils onto the emergent writing table. It may also be a good idea to put out children's name cards, letters and numbers so that they gain visual reminders of the shapes of letters. Children can then float their bottles in the water.

Extending and varying children's learning
- Provide varied paper and writing materials.
- Each day put a new message from your stooge into the tray.
- Consider sending messages attached to balloons.
- Try and find a 'ship in a bottle' as many children find this fascinating.

3 Forgetful teddy and his letters

Teddy has several letters from his friends, but he keeps losing them. He thinks that if he knows how many he has got, he will know when he has lost one.

Specific resources
- five letters in envelopes
- crayons
- numbers
- paper
- pencils

Key learning intentions
This activity is designed to help children see the importance of counting and to use numbers as labels.

Links to Foundation Stage curriculum		
Area of learning	**Aspects of learning**	**Curriculum guidance page**
Personal, social and emotional development	Disposition and attitudes Making relationships Behaviour and self-control	32 36 38
Communication, language and literacy	Language for communication	48, 50, 52, 54
Mathematical Development	Numbers as labels and for counting	74
Physical development	Sense of space Movement Using equipment Using tools and materials	104 106, 108 112 114
Creative development	Exploring media and materials	120

Ideas for organising the activity

This activity works well with pairs of children or trios. It is important that children are able to be active and touch the letters. Start by letting the children 'read' teddy's letters. Explain that teddy keeps his letters because he likes having them. Use this as an opportunity for children to talk about letters or cards that are important to them. Tell them that teddy keeps losing his letters and, because he does not know how many he has got, he does not always know if he has lost one.

Ask the children if they could count the letters for teddy. How may are there? Could they find the number that matches? Could they write a note for teddy so that he will know how many he has got?

Extending and varying children's learning

◆ Can the children help teddy think of a safe place where he might put his letters?
◆ Could the children make him a box or decorate a large envelope so that he could put his things together in them?
◆ Vary the number of letters that teddy has according to the 'number' stage of the children.
◆ Play a game where teddy is actually delivering letters. Some are his to keep while others are to be given back to his friends. How many are there now?

4 Sending e-mails and faxes

As well as sending letters, we can also send e-mails and faxes. Would you like to come and look at how this is done?

Specific resources

◆ access to fax machine or e-mail facility, e.g. local public library, school

> **Key learning intentions**
> This activity is designed to encourage children to be interested and aware of ICT. This is an important strand in knowledge and understanding of the world.

Links to Foundation Stage curriculum		
Area of learning	**Aspects of learning**	**Curriculum guidance page**
Personal, social and emotional development	Disposition and attitudes Making relationships Behaviour and self-control	32 36 38
Communication, language and literacy	Language for communication Language for thinking	48, 50, 52, 54 56–8
Mathematical development	Numbers as labels and for counting Calculating Shape, space and measures	74 76 78–80
Knowledge and understanding of the world	Exploration and investigation Information and communication technology	86, 88 92
Physical development	Movement Using equipment Using tools and materials	106, 108 112 114

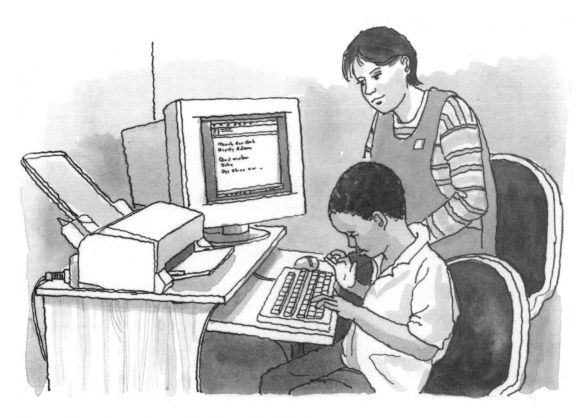

Encourage them to do as much as possible of the pressing of buttons

Ideas for organising the activity

This activity needs to be carried out with individual children or pairs so that they can participate and easily see what is happening. Where possible, agree a time with the recipient of the e-mail or fax so that they can send a response back quickly.

Begin by telling children that as well as sending messages in letters and postcards, some people send messages in other ways. Ask the children if they can think of a message that they would like to send to the recipient. Encourage them to do as much as possible of the pressing of buttons.

Extending and varying children's learning

◆ Provide mock computers or fax machines for children to use in the role-play area.
◆ If possible, continue the link between the recipient and the children.
◆ Show the children examples of Braille to show other ways in which people send messages.
◆ Take photographs of the activity and use these as prompts to encourage children to recall the activity later.

5 Delivering letters

Let's play a delivery game. Here are some boxes, parcels and letters that need taking to different parts of the outdoor play area. You might use your tricycle, pram, or just walk on the chalk lines to the delivery area.

Specific resources

- wrapped parcels
- large boxes to act as delivery points
- tricycles, prams, pushchairs, if available
- other outdoor equipment such as cones, play tunnels, if available
- padded envelopes
- chalk lines

Key learning intentions

This activity encourages children's locomotive and gross motor skills. It should also encourage greater spatial awareness.

Links to Foundation Stage curriculum

Area of learning	Aspects of learning	Curriculum guidance page
Personal, social and emotional development	Disposition and attitudes Self-confidence and self-esteem	32 34
Communication, language and literacy	Language for communication Language for thinking Handwriting	48, 50, 52, 54 56–8 66
Mathematical development	Shape, space and measures	78–80
Knowledge and understanding of the world	Exploration and investigation	86, 88
Physical development	Using tools and materials Sense of space Movement	114 104 106, 108
Creative development	Imagination	124

Ideas for organising the activity

This activity should be done outdoors if possible. (It can be done indoors, although it may not be possible to put down any chalk lines.) Draw some wiggly chalk lines for children to follow around the play area. At the start of the wiggly line, there should be some parcels, letters, etc. in a box, and at the end of the line another box where the children can put them. Give the children the idea of how they may enjoy delivering the packets. If possible, put out play tunnels, hoops and other equipment, which will encourage the children to move in a variety of ways.

During the activity, model the use of positional language, e.g. 'I think that this line finishes *behind* the bench.' Many children will want to develop this activity into role play, so it may be an idea to provide dressing-up props as well.

Extending and varying children's learning

◆ Encourage the children to make the parcels and 'write' the letters for this activity.
◆ Give the children chalk so that they can use it to elaborate the chalk lines.
◆ Consider having some packets or parcels that require children to work together to deliver them.

6 Making our own writing paper and envelopes

Look at all this lovely stationery that is used for writing notes and letters. Would you like to make your own so that you can use it?

Specific resources

◆ decorated envelopes and writing paper to use as examples
◆ stickers
◆ ink stamps
◆ ribbons
◆ scissors
◆ gummed paper
◆ sequins
◆ magazines
◆ glue

Key learning intentions
This activity will encourage children's imagination and creative skills. This activity should also prompt some children to write.

Links to Foundation Stage curriculum		
Area of learning	**Aspects of learning**	**Curriculum guidance page**
Personal, social and emotional development	Disposition and attitudes Behaviour and self-control	32 38
Communication, language and literacy	Language for communication Language for thinking Writing	48, 50, 52, 54 56–8 64
Mathematical development	Numbers as labels and for counting	74
Knowledge and understanding of the world	Exploration and investigation	86, 88
Physical development	Using tools and materials	114
Creative development	Exploring media and materials Imagination	120 124

Ideas for organising the activity

This activity will work well with small groups of children. Begin by talking to children about letters, cards or party invitations that they have received. Do they notice the pictures and patterns? Show children a selection of different writing papers and ask children if they would like to make their own. Encourage children to think about who they might like to send a letter to. For this activity to be a creative one, it is important that children should be free to explore their own ideas – even if they may not conform to our usual ideas of what note paper might look like.

Extending and varying children's learning

◆ Set up an emergent writing table where children can go to write on their note paper. Consider having real stamps and encouraging children to post their letters.

◆ Put out a range of birthday cards. Can children find their favourite ones? Can they identify how old the child will be?

◆ Children can make birthday cards for each other as well as teddy and other favourite characters.

◆ Collect and show children 'old' letters that have been sent. Can they see that the paper has faded or that ink was used rather than biro or pencil?

Theme 12 Parties

Parties are usually important and exciting events in young children's lives. This theme can act as a starting point for having your own party in the setting – and finding something to celebrate!

Inside the box on each area of learning below is a range of ideas for activities and stories on the theme of parties. You will find on the following pages a ready-made activity plan for the first idea listed in each box. In addition, all the stories mentioned are listed in the Booklist on pages 250–252.

Ideas to suggest to parents
- ◆ Point out different types of cards and invitations when they are out shopping.
- ◆ Talk to their child about parties and celebrations that are important in their family.
- ◆ Show their child photographs of celebrations that they have been to.
- ◆ Show their child different types of clothes that might be worn to parties.

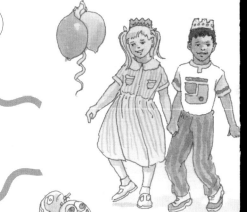

Personal, social and emotional development
- ◆ *Activity plan: Making and wrapping presents (p. 160)*
- ◆ Display: How old are you?
- ◆ Teddy activity – no one will come to his party.
- ◆ Stories:
  - ◆ *Alfie and the Birthday Surprise*
  - ◆ *Spot Goes to the Party*
  - ◆ *Worried Arthur and the Birthday Party*

Communication, language and literacy
- ◆ *Activity plan: Pass the feely parcel (p. 161)*
- ◆ Sorting tray – which objects begin with the letter 'p'?
- ◆ Make place names for the table.
- ◆ Write some party invitations to members of staff, parents and others.
- ◆ Drawing letters and shapes in trays of dry coloured rice (see p. 197).
- ◆ Stories:
  - ◆ *Frog and a Very Special Day*
  - ◆ *My Present*
  - ◆ *Nicky and the Fantastic Birthday Gift*
  - ◆ *Pass the jam Jim*
  - ◆ *Spot Bakes a Cake*
  - ◆ *Worried Arthur and the Birthday Party*

Creative development

* *Activity plan: Make a party hat (p. 166)*
* Musical bumps.
* Role-play area: Parties for the dolls, teddies and other cuddly toys.
* Musical statues.
* Party blowers – how loud and how soft can you make them?
* Make a dough cake and decorate with buttons.

Physical development

* *Activity plan: Name game treasure hunt (p. 165)*
* Hunt the thimble (or other object).
* Circle game – call out the name of another child and roll the ball to them.
* Sleeping lions.
* Making and playing with confetti.
* Pack a party bag.
* Balloons – blow them up and then let them go!
* Bubbles – chase the bubbles.
* Keep the balloon in the air.

Knowledge and understanding of the world

* *Activity plan: Parties that I have been to (p. 164)*
* Making party foods out of malleable materials such as dough and clay.
* Make a jelly – look at the differences.

Mathematical development

* *Activity plan: Make quatre, quatre cakes (p. 163)*
* Laying out a party table – match each plate with a cup and a napkin.
* Making paper chains (with a pattern, e.g. red, blue, red, blue).
* Look at the birthday card – now put the number of candles on the cake.
* How old are you?
* How many items in the party bag – one, two, three or more?

Activity plans for the theme 'parties'

1 Making and wrapping presents

Specific resources
- crayons
- paper
- scissors
- sticky tape
- tissue paper
- boxes
- 'treasures' such as a feather, bead, marble, piece of fabric, shell

---

Key learning intentions

The aim of this activity is to help children enjoy giving and thinking about others. It should also encourage children to talk about presents, as well as developing their hand-eye co-ordination and their imagination.

Links to Foundation Stage curriculum

Area of learning	Aspects of learning	Curriculum guidance page
Personal, social and emotional development	Disposition and attitudes Self-confidence and self-esteem Sense of community	32 34 42
Communication, language and literacy	Language for communication Language for thinking	48, 50, 52, 54 56–8
Mathematical development	Numbers as labels and for counting Calculating Shape, space and measures	74 76 78–80
Physical development	Using equipment Using tools and materials	112 114
Creative development	Imagination	124

Ideas for organising the activity

This activity works well with small groups, although you may wish to work with individuals or pairs of children if they need extra support.

Put a box of 'treasures' out so that children can touch and play with them (small items that can be easily wrapped, but hold children's attention, e.g. pearl buttons, feathers, shells, strips of lace). Tell them that sometimes very small things make lovely presents. They have to think of someone who they would like to give a 'treasure' to.

Children then have to think about how to wrap or box their gift and how to decorate it. Ideally, this should be a creative activity, so the role of the adult is that of support rather than direction. Use this as an opportunity to talk about receiving and giving presents and also things that make us feel happy. Encourage children to 'write' their own special message to the person.

Extending and varying children's learning

◆ Put out paper, sticky tape, small boxes and crayons as part of the role-play area so that children can recreate this play.
◆ Build up a box of treasures that can be used for other occasions.
◆ Using paints, help children to make their own wrapping paper.
◆ Put out cards, envelopes and crayons so that children can make and 'write' their own cards.

---

2 Pass the feely parcel

This is like 'pass the parcel', but when the music stops, you have to guess what is inside by feeling it.

Specific resources

◆ several parcels with everyday objects inside, e.g. pencil, ball, book

---

Key learning intentions
This activity is designed to help children learn to ask questions and to expand their vocabulary. They will also be learning to co-operate with others and listen carefully.

Links to Foundation Stage curriculum

Area of learning	Aspects of learning	Curriculum guidance page
Personal, social and emotional development	Disposition and attitudes Making relationships	32 36
Communication, language and literacy	Language for communication Language for thinking	48, 50, 52, 54 56–8
Mathematical development	Numbers as labels and for counting Shape, space and measures	74 78–80
Knowledge and understanding of the world	Exploration and investigation Information and communication technology Sense of time	86, 88 92 94
Physical development	Movement Using tools and materials	106, 108 114
Creative development	Exploring media and materials Music Imagination	120 122 124

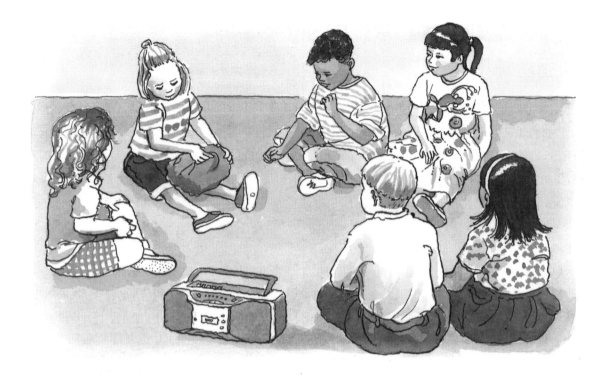

Encourage the children to talk about how the parcel feels and why they are making their guess

Ideas for organising the activity

This activity works well with between five and eight children. Larger numbers will not work as well, as children are likely to become bored if they are waiting for the parcel. Find out which children have played 'pass the parcel' – can they remember how to play the game?

Tell the children that the parcel is passed around the circle when the music is playing. When the music stops, the child with the parcel has to feel the parcel and guess what is inside. To extend children's language, encourage the children to talk about the way the parcel feels and why they are making their guess. With younger children or with children whose language skills are not fully developed, you may need to model the language first with a stooge, e.g. 'Now teddy, what do you think is inside? Teddy, what does it feel like? Is it soft, round or hard?'

You can also use this as an opportunity to count the number of parcels that have been prepared and to count the number of children playing the game.

Extending and varying children's learning

◆ Groups of children can find and wrap up objects in preparation for the game.
◆ Objects can be put in boxes, which the children have to rattle.
◆ Make up a song to sing while the parcel is going around.
◆ Encourage children to stop and start the tape recorder (this covers the ICT aspect of learning in 'Knowledge and understanding of the world').
◆ Encourage children to recreate this game in their role play by putting out the things they may need to make and use the parcels.
◆ Sort wrapped objects into hard or soft, round or square, with pairs of children.

3 Make quatre, quatre cakes $=^+_\times^-$

Let's make some cakes for our party. This recipe uses a balance rather than kitchen scales.

Specific resources

- balancing scales
- eggs
- self-raising flour
- oven
- sugar
- soft margarine
- bun tins or paper cake cases

Key learning intentions

This activity helps children to count, weigh and measure. It also helps to develop hand-eye co-ordination and to learn about personal hygiene.

Links to Foundation Stage curriculum

Area of learning	Aspects of learning	Curriculum guidance page
Personal, social and emotional development	Disposition and attitudes Self-care	32 40
Communication, language and literacy	Language for communication Language for thinking	48, 50, 52, 54 56–8
Mathematical development	Numbers as labels and for counting Calculating Shape, space and measures	74 76 78–80
Physical development	Using equipment	112

Ideas for organising the activity

This cooking activity is ideal for children because they can weigh and measure the ingredients for themselves. The cake mixture is virtually identical to a fairy cake or Victoria sponge mixture. It is best carried out with individual children or pairs so that they can be active at all times.

Take one egg and put it on the scales. Ask the children to put in enough margarine so that it balances with the egg. The margarine is then put into the mixing bowl. The sugar is then weighed in the same way and mixed with the margarine. Finally the self-raising flour is weighed so that it balances with the egg and they are both put in the mixing bowl. The children then put spoonfuls of the mixture into either paper cases or bun tins. The adult should put the cakes into an oven (gas mark 4 or 180°C) for 12–15 minutes or until golden brown and firm to the touch. Using one egg, the mixture should produce about eight fairy cakes.

During the cooking process, refer to culinary utensils by name so that children's vocabulary is increased. They should also be asked to talk about what they are doing and the changes they can see in the mixture.

Health and safety

As with any cooking activity, it is important to check that children do not have special dietary needs. Good hygiene should be maintained and children should be kept away from the oven.

Extending and varying children's learning

◆ Children can decorate their finished cakes.
◆ Children can 'write' out their own recipe.
◆ Encourage children to use the balancing scales by putting them in the role-play area.
◆ Ask children to make 'pretend' cakes using dough.
◆ Using photos, ask the children to correctly sequence this activity.
◆ Read stories about cooking, e.g. *The Gingerbread Man, Spot Bakes a Cake* by Eric Hill.

4 Parties that I have been to

Specific resources

◆ wrapping paper
◆ party hats
◆ birthday cards
◆ New Year cards
◆ photos the children have brought in
◆ photos or cuttings of parties from magazines
◆ balloons
◆ streamers
◆ wedding invitations
◆ party food
◆ drawings the children have made

Key learning intentions
This activity should help children talk about parties that have special importance for them and their families or communities. This activity should also encourage hand-eye co-ordination as children should be involved with putting up the display.

Links to Foundation Stage curriculum

Area of learning	Aspects of learning	Curriculum guidance page
Personal, social and emotional development	Disposition and attitudes Self-confidence and self-esteem Making relationships Sense of community	32 34 36 42
Communication, language and literacy	Language for communication Language for thinking Linking sounds with letters Reading Writing Handwriting	48, 50, 52, 54 56–8 60 62 64 66
Mathematical development	Shape, space and measures	78–80
Knowledge and understanding of the world	Exploration and investigation Designing and making skills Sense of time Sense of place Cultures and beliefs	86, 88 90 94 96 98

▽

Physical development	Using equipment	112
	Using tools and materials	114
Creative development	Exploring media and materials	120
	Responding to experiences, and	
	expressing and communicating ideas	126

Ideas for organising the activity

Start by talking to pairs or very small groups of children about parties. You may show them photos of parties in books or magazines. Ask them about any parties they remember going to. Was it a long time ago? What did they do? Who was there? The discussion can be widened out to parties in families, e.g. weddings, festivals, birthdays. Bring out a selection of party objects for children to look at, e.g. balloons, streamers and cards. Ask them to choose which ones might be displayed.

Encourage children to cut up photos in magazines that they can use for the display as well as asking parents if there are any photos that can be brought it. Ask them to make things for the display, e.g. 'write' their own invitations, draw pictures of parties.

When putting up the display, consider using wrapping paper as a backing and then putting on drawings, photos and also objects such as streamers and cards. Encourage children to write their own captions and labels.

Extending and varying children's learning

◆ Ask children to make their own party book – using photos they have brought in.
◆ Paint pictures of party foods.
◆ In pairs, encourage children to talk about party food that they enjoy.

5 Name game treasure hunt

Someone has hidden all your names. Can you and your partner find your names?

Specific resources

◆ laminated name cards or pieces of paper with the children's names on them

---

Key learning intentions
Children will gain spatial awareness and searching skills whilst building letter recognition skills.

Links to Foundation Stage curriculum

Area of learning	Aspects of learning	Curriculum guidance page
Personal, social and emotional development	Disposition and attitudes	32
	Making relationships	36
	Behaviour and self-control	38
	Self-care	40

▽

Communication, language and literacy	Language for communication Language for thinking Linking sounds with letters Reading	48, 50, 52, 54 56–8 60 62
Mathematical development	Shape, space and measures	78–80
Knowledge and understanding of the world	Exploration and investigation Sense of place	86, 88 96
Physical development	Sense of space Movement	104 106, 108

Ideas for organising the activity

Hide the children's names either in or out of doors. With younger children you may need to add a picture to their name so that they can recognise it more easily, or pair up an older child with a younger one. Ask them if they can find their names in pairs. The key to this activity is to adapt it according to the children's needs.

You can, for example, produce several names for each child so that they have more opportunities to recognise it. They can also be helped by carrying an example of their own name, so that they can look at a name and then see if it matches. After the activity, ask children to say where they found their name – encourage the use of positional language, e.g. 'in front of', 'up', 'across from'. This game tends to be very popular, with children wanting to repeat it several times!

Extending and varying children's learning

◆ Children can take it in turns to hide each other's names.
◆ Encourage children to recreate this game in the role-play area by providing them with strips of paper and pencils so that they can 'write' names.
◆ Children can look for each other's names.
◆ Initial letters only of the children's names are hidden.

---

6 Make a party hat

Let's make a party hat – perhaps we can also make one or two for some of the members of staff as well. What type of things would you like to have on your hat?

Specific resources

◆ strips of paper   ◆ stapler   ◆ sequins   ◆ feathers
◆ beads   ◆ crayons   ◆ other materials to decorate

> **Key learning intentions**
> This activity will help children to use their design skills and use a range of textures creatively.

Links to Foundation Stage curriculum		
Area of learning	**Aspects of learning**	**Curriculum guidance page**
Personal, social and emotional development	Disposition and attitudes Making relationships Self-care	32 36 40
Communication, language and literacy	Language for communication Language for thinking Writing Handwriting	48, 50, 52, 54 56–8 64 66
Mathematical development	Shape, space and measures	78–80
Knowledge and understanding of the world	Exploration and investigation Designing and making skills	86, 88 90
Physical development	Using equipment Using tools and materials	112 114
Creative development	Exploring media and materials Responding to experiences, and expressing and communicating ideas	120 126

Ideas for organising the activity

With pairs or small groups of children, show them how, using a strip of paper and a stapler, a crown can be made, which can form the basis of a hat. Encourage the children to practise using the stapler (under supervision) before asking them to choose the materials that they would like to use to make their own hat. For this activity to be a creative one, children should be supported, but not directed, even if their choice of materials is obscure!

Using questions, help children to work out how large the band of the hat needs to be, e.g. 'Is it too small or too big?' Ask them to find a way of making 'their mark' on the hat. Some children may attempt to write their name, others may draw a symbol.

Extending and varying children's learning

◆ Encourage children to make more hats to fit different sizes, e.g. a doll, teddy.
◆ Use the materials that have held children's attention to produce a collage.
◆ Take photographs of the process of making hats and ask children later to sequence them in order.

Theme 13 Animals

Most young children have seen cats, dogs and other pets, even if they do not own any. This theme is a good starting point for looking at animals and caring for them. Make sure children pick up the message that animals are not playthings and that they need caring for properly.

Inside the box on each area of learning below is a range of ideas for activities and stories on the theme of animals. You will find on the following pages a ready-made activity plan for the first idea listed in each box. In addition, all the stories mentioned are listed in the Booklist on pages 250–252.

Ideas to suggest to parents

◆ Point out dogs, cats, birds and other animals that their child may see.

◆ Talk to their child about the different features of dogs, e.g. shaggy, large, pointed ears.

◆ Point out to their child foods and materials for pets, e.g. in the supermarket or in the pet shop.

Personal, social and emotional development

◆ *Activity plan: Animal happy families (p. 170)*

◆ Display: Our pets.

◆ Losing a pet.

◆ Visitors to talk about pets, e.g. RSPCA, Guide Dogs for the Blind.

◆ Bring and buy sale for RSPCA.

◆ Stories:
  ◆ *John Brown, Rose and the Midnight Cat* – sharing.
  ◆ *Six Dinner Sid*

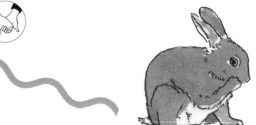

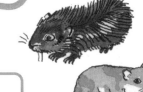

Communication, language and literacy

◆ *Activity plan: I am thinking of a pet (p. 171)*

◆ Stories:
  ◆ *The Cats of Tiffany Street*
  ◆ *Dear Zoo*
  ◆ *Flea's Best Friend*
  ◆ *I Want a Pet*
  ◆ *My Cat*
  ◆ *Prowlpuss*
  ◆ *Six Dinner Sid*
  ◆ *Topsy and Tim and the New Puppy*
  ◆ *Topsy and Tim Look After Their Pets*

◆ Picture lotto – can you match the animals?

◆ Pairs – baby and mother.

◆ Same and different – photos of different breeds of dogs, cats.

◆ Same and different – cuddly toys.

◆ Mog the forgetful cat.

◆ Role-play area: Vets.

◆ Name the pet (could be a cuddly toy).

Creative development

◆ *Activity plan: Find your partner – animal sounds (p. 176)*

◆ Music: Saint Saens' *Carnival of Animals* – can you move like the animals?

◆ Song: 'Bobby Bingo, There was a farmer who had a dog and Bingo was his name – o'

◆ Make a shoebox home for a pet.

Physical development

◆ *Activity plan: Take the pet to the vet (p. 175)*

◆ Water – with animals, farms.

◆ Sand – make a home for these animals.

◆ Slides and obstacle course.

◆ Slide, hop or run? I'll call one out. Can you do it?

◆ What's the time, Mr Wolf?

◆ Parachute game – listen to the name of the animal and run into the middle if yours is called.

Knowledge and understanding of the world

◆ *Activity plan: Pet masks (p. 173)*

◆ What animals can we find outdoors?

◆ Match the food to the pet, e.g. cat food, dog food, bird seed.

◆ Where does my pet sleep?

◆ Which animal made this print?

◆ Bug box – what can you see in here?

◆ Make a birdseed cake.

◆ Visit by a vet.

Mathematical development

◆ *Activity plan: Animals in the sand pit (p. 172)*

◆ Make an animal game – roll the dice and put in the part.

◆ Put the animals into pairs – are there any without a partner?

◆ Which cuddly toy will fit into this box?

◆ Sorting cuddly toys according to size.

◆ Pictogram – which pets do you have or would you like?

◆ How many hidden animals can you see in this picture?

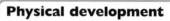

Activity plans for the theme 'animals'

I Animal happy families

Come and play this fun game. Can you make a family out of these cards?

Specific resources

◆ cards, which have pictures of animals on them, e.g. four cards with cats, four cards with dogs, four cards with rabbits, etc.

Key learning intentions

This activity will help children to take turns and build relationships with others in the setting, while also helping them to match.

Links to Foundation Stage curriculum

Area of learning	Aspects of learning	Curriculum guidance page
Personal, social and emotional development	Disposition and attitudes Self-confidence and self-esteem Making relationships Behaviour and self-control Self-care Sense of community	32 34 36 38 40 42
Communication, language and literacy	Language for communication Language for thinking Reading	48, 50, 52, 54 56–8 62
Mathematical development	Numbers as labels and for counting	74
Knowledge and understanding of the world	Exploration and investigation Sense of time Cultures and beliefs	86, 88 94 98
Physical development	Movement Using tools and materials	106, 108 114
Creative development	Imagination	124

Ideas for organising the activity

This activity works well with pairs of children at first, then small groups if they are able to co-operate. Begin by showing children all the animal cards. Can they group the cards according to families? Give them a different card each and put the rest of the cards face down. Ask them to take it in turns to turn over a card and see if it is part of their family. If not, they put it face down again.

Use this activity as an opportunity for children to talk about their families.

Extending and varying children's learning

◆ Encourage children to make their own animal family games by cutting out pictures of animals and putting them onto card.

◆ Older children can play the equivalent of happy families by holding cards and asking others if they have one of their family members.
◆ Play a 'roll a dice' game with children taking the number of cards shown on the dice – how many pets have they got?
◆ Use cards to play a game where one child describes the card that they are looking at – the other children have to point to the card they are describing.

2 I am thinking of a pet

Let's play a game with our toy animals. I will describe a pet – can you work out which one it is?

Specific resources

◆ cuddly toys   ◆ paper   ◆ drawing materials

Key learning intentions
This activity is designed for children to extend their descriptive vocabulary and give them opportunities to practise using questions.

Links to Foundation Stage curriculum		
Area of learning	**Aspects of learning**	**Curriculum guidance page**
Personal, social and emotional development	Disposition and attitudes Making relationships Behaviour and self-control Self-care Sense of community	32 36 38 40 42
Communication, language and literacy	Language for communication Language for thinking Linking sounds with letters Reading Writing	48, 50, 52, 54 56–8 60 62 64
Mathematical development	Numbers as labels and for counting Shape, space and measures	74 78–80
Knowledge and understanding of the world	Exploration and investigation Designing and making skills	86, 88 90
Physical development	Using tools and materials	114
Creative development	Exploring media and materials Imagination Responding to experiences, and expressing and communicating ideas	120 124 126

Ideas for organising the activity

This activity works well with small groups of children. Put out a selection of different cuddly toys and plastic animals on a table or in the centre of where children are sitting. Tell the children that you will describe an animal and they can take it in turns to go and pick up the animal that you have in mind.

Model language such as 'furry', 'soft', 'plastic', etc. For children who are beginning to notice letter sounds, give the initial sound of the animal or a word with which it rhymes, e.g. 'It rhymes with log and begins with a 'd'.' Once you have played the game a few times, ask children if they could describe an animal for the others to guess.

Extending and varying children's learning

- Put out some cardboard boxes so that positional language can be used, e.g. 'on top of' 'underneath'.
- Ask children to sort the animals out according to their sizes or type.
- Leave the animals out so that children can recreate this game for themselves.

3 Animals in the sand pit

Look at the sand pit today – if you scoop you may find some animals.

Specific resources

- scoops
- boxes
- pencils
- paper
- numbers on cards from 1–5
- hand-held vacuum cleaner or dustpan and brush
- plastic animals – farm animals, dinosaurs, snakes, or whatever is available
- sand, either in a small tray or in a large container

Key learning intentions

The aim of this activity is to encourage children to use numbers as labels, to compare groups of objects and also to sort.

Links to Foundation Stage curriculum

Area of learning	Aspects of learning	Curriculum guidance page
Personal, social and emotional development	Disposition and attitudes Self-confidence and self-esteem Making relationships Behaviour and self-control Self-care	32 34 36 38 40
Communication, language and literacy	Language for communication Language for thinking Writing Handwriting	48, 50, 52, 54 56–8 64 66

Mathematical development	Numbers as labels and for counting Calculating Shape, space and measures	74 76 78–80
Knowledge and understanding of the world	Exploration and investigation Information and communication technology	86, 88 92
Physical development	Movement Using tools and materials	106, 108 114
Creative development	Exploring media and materials Imagination	120 124

Ideas for organising the activity

This activity works well with pairs or individual children so that they can be active at all times. Begin by asking them if they can find the hidden plastic animals in the sand. As they are finding the animals, encourage them to count what they have found.

Once most or all of the animals have been found, ask the children if they can put them into groups to sort them out. Boxes or containers can be given to the children to help them separate them. Which group has the most? Which group has the least? If the children are ready to use and recognise numbers, ask them if they can find the number that matches each group. Encourage them to hide the animals again for each other and to play the game again.

Extending and varying children's learning

◆ Leave the animals, the boxes and other objects out so that children can recreate this play.
◆ Encourage children to 'write' their own numbers and put them in the boxes.
◆ Give each child several animals – when they roll the dice they must bury the number shown back in the sand pit – the dice can be altered to only show 1, 2 and 3.
◆ Ask the children if they would like to create sand homes for the animals.

4 Pet masks

Can you make a mask of a pet? A rabbit, dog, cat, or even a hamster, perhaps?

Specific resources

◆ card
◆ stapler
◆ markers
◆ scissors
◆ crayons
◆ wool
◆ glue
◆ elastic
◆ other materials available

Key learning intentions
This activity is designed to encourage children's designing and making skills. They will also gain confidence in using tools.

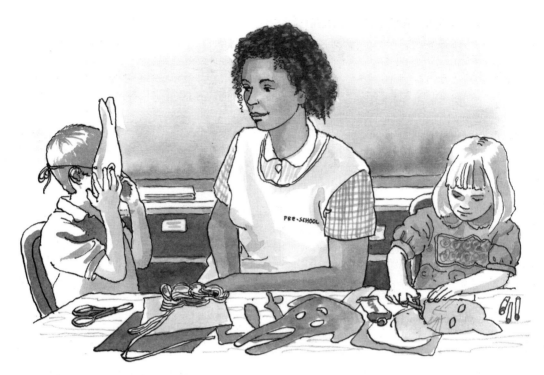

This activity helps give children confidence in using tools

Links to Foundation Stage curriculum		
Area of learning	**Aspects of learning**	**Curriculum guidance page**
Personal, social and emotional development	Disposition and attitudes Self-confidence and self-esteem Making relationships Behaviour and self-control Self-care	32 34 36 38 40
Communication, language and literacy	Language for communication Language for thinking Handwriting	48, 50, 52, 54 56–8 66
Mathematical development	Shape, space and measures	78–80
Knowledge and understanding of the world	Exploration and investigation Designing and making skills Cultures and beliefs	86, 88 90 98
Physical development	Sense of space Movement Using tools and materials	104 106, 108 114
Creative development	Exploring media and materials Imagination Responding to experiences, and expressing and communicating ideas	120 124 126

Ideas for organising the activity

This activity works best with pairs of children as significant adult support will be required. Begin by showing children the materials that are available and also some photos or pictures of pets. Show them how they can make a mask by using a paper plate and cutting out eyes and a nose, or if they do not want something over their faces they can add some ears to a band of card.

Once you have shown children different ways of making a mask, encourage them to think about what they would like to do. The role of the adult in this activity is to be supportive rather than directive. This means following children's suggestions and giving them ideas to make them work.

Extending and varying children's learning

◆ Put some music on so that children can pretend to be their animal.
◆ Encourage the children to write their own names on their masks.
◆ Ask children if they know what their pet would need to eat.
◆ Ask children if they know when their pet goes to bed – is it a nocturnal animal?

5 Take the pet to the vet

Let's pretend that your cuddly animal is ill. You will need to take it to the vet!

Specific resources

◆ equipment such as play tunnels, slides, tricycles, wheel barrows
◆ chalk   ◆ cuddly toys   ◆ cat baskets (if possible)

> **Key learning intentions**
> This activity is designed to promote children's sense of movement, locomotive and gross motor skills.

Links to Foundation Stage curriculum		
Area of learning	**Aspects of learning**	**Curriculum guidance page**
Personal, social and emotional development	Disposition and attitudes Behaviour and self-control Self-care	32 38 40
Communication, language and literacy	Handwriting	66
Mathematical development	Shape, space and measures	78–80
Knowledge and understanding of the world	Designing and making skills Sense of place	90 96
Physical development	Sense of space Movement Using equipment Using tools and materials	104 106, 108 112 114

▽

Creative development	Exploring media and materials	120
	Imagination	124
	Responding to experiences, and expressing and communicating ideas	126

Ideas for organising the activity

This activity can be carried out with small groups of children – up to about eight. Begin by setting out an obstacle-type course using the equipment you have available. Include a chalk line road, if possible, which leads to the vets. This can be just a chalked out square or a walled part of the outdoor area or room.

Ask each child to choose a cuddly toy. Tell them that their 'pet' is poorly and needs to be seen by a vet – can they take their pet to the vet?

Use this activity to model positional language such as 'up', 'behind', 'under', etc. Encourage the children to draw their own chalk roads to the vets.

Extending and varying children's learning

- ◆ Can children draw a 'map' showing the way to the vets?
- ◆ Encourage children to build a vets' practice using boxes.
- ◆ Encourage children to design their own obstacle course.

6 Find your partner – animal sounds

Can you walk around and make your animal sound? Can you find other children making the same sound?

Specific resources

- ◆ pictures of pets or farm animals

Key learning intentions

This activity will help children explore sounds as well as to use their imagination.

Links to Foundation Stage curriculum

Area of learning	Aspects of learning	Curriculum guidance page
Personal, social and emotional development	Disposition and attitudes Making relationships Behaviour and self-control Self-care Sense of community	32 36 38 40 42
Communication, language and literacy	Language for communication Language for thinking Linking sounds with letters	48, 50, 52, 54 56–8 60
Knowledge and understanding of the world	Sense of place Cultures and beliefs	96 98

▽

Physical development	Sense of space	104
	Movement	106, 108
Creative development	Exploring media and materials	120
	Imagination	124
	Responding to experiences, and expressing and communicating ideas	126

Ideas for organising the activity

This activity works well with groups of children. Prepare several pictures of animals so that there is more than one animal type. Begin the activity by asking children if they can make any animal noises. Show the children the pictures or cards of animals – can they make the sounds of the animal shown? Use this as an opportunity to check that they know the names of the animals. Once they are ready, begin the game. Give each child a picture of an animal and ask the children to go around the room making the sound of the animal until they have found a partner or their group.

Extending and varying children's learning

◆ Encourage older children's reading by writing the name of the animal alongside a picture on the card.
◆ Ask children if they would like to make animal masks.
◆ Encourage children to move like the animals represented on their cards.

Theme 14 Potatoes

This theme is a good starting point as most families eat potatoes in some form or another. Children will be able to talk about their favourite ways of eating potatoes. Potatoes are robust objects and children should be able to touch and play with them. Most settings should also be able to carry out one or more cooking activities using potatoes, as they can be cooked in a microwave. From this starting point, you may wish to consider looking at different types of vegetables.

Inside the box on each area of learning below is a range of ideas for activities and stories on the theme of potatoes. You will find on the following pages a ready-made activity plan for the first idea listed in each box. In addition, all the stories mentioned are listed in the Booklist on pages 250–252.

Ideas to suggest to parents

◆ Point out different fruit and vegetables that they eat at home.
◆ Encourage their child to look at the range of fruit and vegetables in the supermarket or in the greengrocers.
◆ Encourage their child to taste a new vegetable.

Personal, social and emotional development

◆ *Activity plan: Planting and growing potatoes (p. 180)*
◆ Display: This is how we eat our potatoes.
◆ My favourite foods.
◆ Tasting potatoes cooked in a variety of ways – which one do you prefer?

Communication, language and literacy

◆ *Activity plan: What has teddy got? (p. 181)*
◆ Rhyme: 'One potato, two potatoes, three potatoes more ...'
◆ Stories:
    ◆ *The Great Big Enormous Turnip*
    ◆ *Oliver's Vegetables*
◆ Feely bag: Guess the vegetable.
◆ Display of objects beginning with the letter sound 'p'.
◆ Role-play area: Fish and chip shop.

Creative development

◆ *Activity plan: Observational drawing/painting of potatoes (p. 186)*

◆ Potato printing and rolling potatoes in paint to make marks.

◆ Role-play area: Fruit and vegetable shop.

◆ Making a potato head.

Physical development

◆ *Activity plan: New, boiled and mashed – a parachute game (p. 185)*

◆ Making mashed potatoes.

◆ Potato and spoon obstacle course.

◆ Catching and rolling games – hot potato.

◆ Hunt the hidden potatoes in the outdoor area.

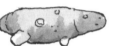
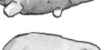
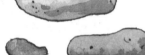
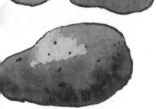
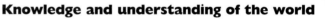

Knowledge and understanding of the world

◆ *Activity plan: Delivering a potato (p. 183)*

◆ Can you make a boat to stop my potato from getting wet?

◆ Do you eat potatoes? Mashed, fried, sweet potatoes or boiled?

◆ Let's make jacket potatoes for lunch in the microwave.

◆ What are your favourite vegetables?

◆ Can you sort out those vegetables that grow in the ground?

Mathematical development

◆ *Activity plan: Rolling potatoes (p. 182)*

◆ Grouping potatoes – white or red.

◆ How many baby potatoes to balance this baking potato?

◆ Ordering potatoes according to size.

◆ Weighing potatoes.

◆ How many potatoes will fit in this bag?

◆ Can you find a potato that is too large for your hand?

◆ Feely bag: How many potatoes can you feel – one, two, three or four?

Activity plans for the theme 'potatoes'

I Planting and growing potatoes

Can we plant our own potatoes and see what happens?

Specific resources
◆ seed potatoes (if possible) otherwise potatoes that are beginning to sprout
◆ containers   ◆ sticky labels

Key learning intentions
This activity is designed to help children care for their environment and take some responsibility. It will also help them to observe and find out about living and growing things.

Links to Foundation Stage curriculum

Area of learning	Aspects of learning	Curriculum guidance page
Personal, social and emotional development	Disposition and attitudes Making relationships Behaviour and self-control Self-care	32 36 38 40
Communication, language and literacy	Language for communication Language for thinking Writing	48, 50, 52, 54 56–8 64
Mathematical development	Shape, space and measures	78–80
Knowledge and understanding of the world	Exploration and investigation Designing and making skills Sense of time	86, 88 90 94
Physical development	Using equipment Using tools and materials	112 114
Creative development	Exploring media and materials	120

Ideas for organising the activity
Bring in a selection of potatoes for pairs or small groups of children to plant. Encourage them to make choices about how to decorate, label and even store their planted potato. Provide sticky labels so that children can 'make' their own mark or write their name.

   Encourage the children to help each other, e.g. holding containers out for each other – this may be an activity where an older child can help a younger one. Make sure that they tidy away after they have finished, e.g. sweeping the floor. They should also wash their hands after handling the potatoes. Measure the potatoes' progress with the children.

Health and safety
If the potatoes are eventually to be harvested, it is important to buy seed potatoes as these should be free of disease.

Extending and varying children's learning

◆ Plant some potatoes in shoeboxes with holes in them so that the roots emerge from the box.
◆ Plant some potatoes outdoors and harvest them.
◆ Observe which potatoes flourish – those planted in sand, water or soil?
◆ Take photographs during the planting process and ask children to sequence them and talk about what they did.

2 What has teddy got?

What has teddy got in his bag? What has he been doing?

Specific resources

◆ fabric bag
◆ potato
◆ pillow case or box
◆ trowel and one other object, e.g. bar of soap
◆ teddy or other soft toy

Key learning intentions
This activity is designed to promote children's overall language development, especially their ability to use language for thinking and for writing.

Links to Foundation Stage curriculum		
Area of learning	**Aspects of learning**	**Curriculum guidance page**
Personal, social and emotional development	Disposition and attitudes Behaviour and self-control	32 38
Communication, language and literacy	Language for communication Language for thinking Writing	48, 50, 52, 54 56–8 64
Mathematical development	Numbers as labels and for counting	74
Knowledge and understanding of the world	Exploration and investigation	86, 88
Physical development	Using tools and materials	114
Creative development	Imagination	124

Ideas for organising the activity

Put the objects in a fabric bag or box. Ask a small group of children to guess what might be in teddy's bag. Take out the objects one by one. Using teddy as a stooge: talk to him about what he has been doing!

Encourage the children to come up with what teddy might have been doing, e.g. 'Teddy has been planting potatoes and now he needs to wash his hands using the soap.' Where possible, try and actually create a story with the children, e.g. 'Once upon a time …' Leave the story bag and the objects out so that children can play and recreate their own story.

Health and safety
Choose objects that you feel will be suitable for children to handle and play with.

Extending and varying children's learning

◆ Vary the objects so that teddy has a new story to tell each day.
◆ Can the children ask teddy questions about what is in his bag?
◆ Write teddy's story out for the children and make it into a book.
◆ Encourage the children to paint or draw teddy's story.
◆ Ask the children if they could 'write' and draw some pictures to help teddy remember what he has been doing.

3 Rolling potatoes

Potatoes come in many different shapes and sizes. Which of these potatoes will roll the furthest?

Specific resources

◆ several potatoes of different shapes including some that are smooth and very rounded

Key learning intentions
This activity is to encourage children to observe the properties of 3D shapes by rolling different shaped potatoes and to observe the differences between potatoes. It should generate some excitement as well as opportunities to develop specific vocabulary.

Links to Foundation Stage curriculum

Area of learning	Aspects of learning	Curriculum guidance page
Personal, social and emotional development	Disposition and attitudes Behaviour and self-control	32 38
Communication, language and literacy	Language for communication Language for thinking	48, 50, 52, 54 56–8
Mathematical development	Shape, space and measures	78–80
Knowledge and understanding of the world	Exploration and investigation	86, 88
Physical development	Using tools and materials	114

Ideas for organising the activity

Bring in a selection of potatoes for small groups or individual children to look at. Ask them to predict which ones would roll. Encourage them to think about why some potatoes roll better than others.

Extending and varying children's learning

◆ Predict the rolling ability of potatoes.
◆ Encourage the children to find ways of measuring and marking out the distances that the potatoes can roll.
◆ Roll other vegetables.
◆ Ask children to make slopes for potatoes to roll down.
◆ Sort potatoes into groups according to how well they roll.
◆ Make obstacle courses for potatoes to roll along.
◆ Compare how well potatoes roll to balls.
◆ Prepare a display of the potatoes that roll well.
◆ Ask the children to draw or make their own recording of the activity.

4 Delivering a potato

Can we deliver this potato from here to there using the remote-controlled truck?

Specific resources

◆ remote-controlled dumper truck or similar toy
◆ small potato to be carried or pulled by the toy

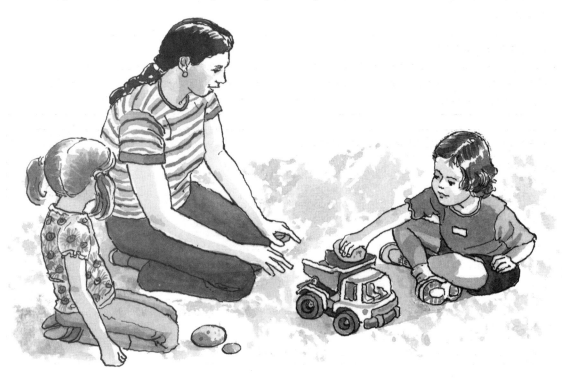

Use prompting questions to help children work out how to use the programmable toy

Key learning intentions

This activity is designed to help children use a programmable toy, which should help them be active when using ICT. Much of the value of this activity lies in the children's exploration and solving of a problem, e.g. calculating how far the truck needs to travel, using positional language.

(If a programmable toy is not available, children could make or adapt vehicles in which to transport a potato, e.g. a train. This would, however, alter the links to the Foundation Stage.)

Links to Foundation Stage curriculum		
Area of learning	**Aspects of learning**	**Curriculum guidance page**
Personal, social and emotional development	Disposition and attitudes Making relationships Behaviour and self-control	32 36 38
Communication, language and literacy	Language for communication Language for thinking	48, 50, 52, 54 56–8
Mathematical development	Numbers as labels and for counting Calculating Shape, space and measures	74 76 78–80
Knowledge and understanding of the world	Exploration and investigation Information and communication technology	86, 88 92
Physical development	Movement Using equipment Using tools and materials	106, 108 112 114

Ideas for organising the activity

This activity needs to be carried out with individual children or pairs, as it tries to encourage them to problem solve and be active in their use of ICT. Adults should use prompting questions to help children work out how best to use the programmable toy. This is an ideal activity for positional language, such as 'in front', 'behind', 'forwards', to be used.

Extending and varying children's learning

◆ Provide obstacles for the remote-controlled toy to manoeuvre around.
◆ Encourage children to draw 'maps' of the route to be taken.
◆ Ask children to make paper roads for the truck to roll on.
◆ Ask the children to draw or make their own recording of the activity.
◆ Take photographs of the activity and use these as prompts to encourage children to recall the activity later.

5 New, boiled and mashed – a parachute game

Each of you is a type of potato. Listen out and move when your name is called.

Specific resources

◆ small parachute if possible, otherwise a sheet or large tablecloth

> **Key learning intentions**
> This activity is designed to help children learn specific vocabulary about potatoes whilst enjoying physical activity with others. Parachute games are very popular with children and can be used in and out of doors.

Links to Foundation Stage curriculum		
Area of learning	**Aspects of learning**	**Curriculum guidance page**
Personal, social and emotional development	Disposition and attitudes Making relationships Behaviour and self-control	32 36 38
Communication, language and literacy	Language for communication	48, 50, 52, 54
Physical development	Sense of space Movement Using equipment Using tools and materials	104 106, 108 112 114
Creative development	Exploring media and materials	120

Ideas for organising the activity

This activity needs to be carried out after children have already 'experienced' potatoes. Gather them around the parachute and give each child one of the following names: 'new', 'boiled' and 'mashed'. With the children, begin shaking the parachute slowly allowing it to rise and fall. Call out one of the names and ask the children with that name to go under the lifted parachute and appear in a new place.

The opportunity to talk about changes to our bodies when exercising should be used as this is one aspect of physical development incorporated into the Foundation Stage.

> **Health and safety**
> To avoid accidents, make sure children do not become over-excited – encourage them to walk at first to their new places, rather than run. Once they become good at finding their way under the parachute, they can speed up.

Extending and varying children's learning

◆ Change the names so that new vocabulary is introduced, e.g. crisps, chips, fries.
◆ Encourage children to run around the outside of the parachute rather than underneath it.
◆ Put potatoes on top of the parachute and see if the children can keep them from rolling off the sides.

6 Observational drawing/painting of potatoes

Teddy wants to show his friend that potatoes can be different. Can we do some drawings/paintings for him to show to his friend?

Specific resources

◆ several potatoes of distinctly different sizes and colours, e.g. new potatoes, sweet potatoes, red potatoes, green potatoes, as well as potatoes which have begun to sprout
◆ drawing and painting materials

Key learning intentions

This activity helps children to express in pictures and marks what they see. Some children may also wish to 'write' about the potatoes. This is essentially a creative activity and adults should take a supportive rather than a directive role.

Links to Foundation Stage curriculum

Area of learning	Aspects of learning	Curriculum guidance page
Personal, social and emotional development	Disposition and attitudes Self-care	32 40
Communication, language and literacy	Language for communication Language for thinking Writing Handwriting	48, 50, 52, 54 56–8 64 66
Knowledge and understanding of the world	Exploration and investigation	86, 88
Physical development	Using equipment Using tools and materials	112 114
Creative development	Exploring media and materials	120

Ideas for organising the activity

Ask the children what makes three potatoes different. Point out differences such as 'eyes' in potatoes, as well as the colours of potatoes. Using a teddy or similar stooge ask children if they could draw or paint a picture for teddy to show his friend.

Encourage the children to express their ' vision' of the potatoes in their own way – do not worry if the final products are not representational. It is important that they learn to draw and paint independently and with confidence.

Extending and varying children's learning

◆ Provide varied textures so that children can use collage techniques.
◆ Provide envelopes and writing paper so that children can 'post' their finished pictures and letters to teddy's friend.
◆ Using a toy telephone, ask the children to talk to teddy's friend about the potatoes.
◆ Make up a potato song with the children about differences in potatoes.

Theme 15 Seeds

This is a good starting point as most children eat seeds in one form or another. You can grow beans and seeds with children so that they can learn about plants. This theme can also be developed into talking about growing, plants, farms and looking at the outside world.

Inside the box on each area of learning below is a range of ideas for activities and stories on the theme of seeds. You will find on the following pages a ready-made activity plan for the first idea listed in each box. In addition, all the stories mentioned are listed in the Booklist on pages 250–252.

Ideas to suggest to parents

◆ Point out seeds, acorns, pods and seedlings.

◆ Grow some cress seeds or a bean at home.

◆ Encourage their child to look after house plants or to water plants in the garden.

Personal, social and emotional development

◆ *Activity plan: Making seed cakes for birds (p. 190)*

◆ Tasting different types of seeds.

◆ Cooking with different seeds – do you use any seeds at home?

◆ Visitor: Keen gardener or allotment society member.

◆ Story: *The Selfish Giant*

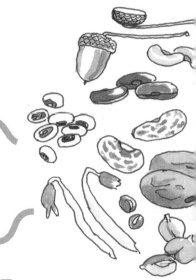

Communication, language and literacy

◆ *Activity plan: Role-play area: Garden centre (p. 191)*

◆ Sequence cards – what happens to the seed, first, second and then third?

◆ Make letter shapes in this tray of sesame seeds.

◆ Stories:
  ◆ *Jack and the Beanstalk*
  ◆ *The Tiny Seed*

◆ Rhymes:
  ◆ 'I had a little nut tree'
  ◆ 'Round and round the garden'

Creative development

- *Activity plan: Paper plate flowers (p. 197)*
- Make a seed collage using seeds, leaves and pasta.
- Drama: Squirrel has found some seeds – where will he hide them?
- Make seed shakers.
- Fruit prints – can you see the seeds?
- Observational drawing of seeds.
- Make your own tray garden for the small world people.

Physical development

- *Activity plan: Find the beans hidden in the rice (p. 195)*
- Use tweezers to pick up large seeds and put them one by one into a small beaker.
- Dough made with seeds inside.
- Water the plants outside.
- Watering cans and buckets.
- Seed mosaic collages.
- Find the beans in the sand tray.

Knowledge and understanding of the world

- *Activity plan: Hunt the beans and seeds (p. 194)*
- Growing seeds – let's look at the changes each day.
- Plant beans – which grows first, indoors or outdoors?
- Where are the seeds inside these fruits?
- What is growing around us at the moment? – Let's go for a walk and see.
- Make a seed packet for teddy to keep his special seeds in.

Mathematical development

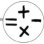

- *Activity plan: Beans in the egg boxes (p. 193)*
- Can you make these seeds balance?
- Which of our sunflower/runner beans will grow the tallest?
- Sorting seeds – smallest to largest.
- Which pile of seeds is the largest?
- Which of these envelopes would be the best for these seeds?
- Make an envelope to fit these seeds in.

I Making seed cakes for birds

Let's make a bird seed cake so that we can feed some birds.

Specific resources

- microwave or saucepan and stove
- lard
- peanuts
- other dried food suitable for birds
- yoghurt pots or similar
- bird seed
- raisins
- 30 cm of string

Key learning intentions

This activity should help children to think about the differences in food tastes that animals, and also people, have. It is also designed to help children to talk and relate to adults.

Links to Foundation Stage curriculum

Area of learning	Aspects of learning	Curriculum guidance page
Personal, social and emotional development	Disposition and attitudes Self-confidence and self-esteem Making relationships Behaviour and self-control Self-care Sense of community	32 34 36 38 40 42
Communication, language and literacy	Language for communication Language for thinking	48, 50, 52, 54 56–8
Mathematical development	Numbers as labels and for counting Calculating Shape, space and measures	74 76 78–80
Knowledge and understanding of the world	Exploration and investigation Designing and making skills Sense of time Sense of place Cultures and beliefs	86, 88 90 94 96 98
Physical development	Sense of space Movement Health and bodily awareness Using equipment Using tools and materials	104 106, 108 110 112 114
Creative development	Imagination Responding to experiences, and expressing and communicating ideas	124 126

Ideas for organising the activity

This activity works best with pairs of children as there is a hot substance involved. Prepare this activity by piercing a hole in the bottom of each yoghurt pot and by cutting the lengths of string. Begin by taking children out of doors. What birds can they see or hear? Show children different types of seeds and let them touch and explore them.

Give each child a bowl and ask them to put a range of seeds inside. Once they have mixed their seeds, they need to make a knot in one end of their length of string and thread it through their yoghurt pot. Encourage them at this point to write on stickers for their pots so that they will recognise them. You will then need to melt the lard. While the children can look at the difference between solid and melted lard, you should take control of melting it and putting some into each of their bowls. They can then stir the seeds into the melted lard. This mixture cools quickly, so they can then spoon the mixture into their yoghurt pot. This needs to be left in a cool place or the fridge to harden. Once hardened, the children can snip the knotted end of the string and turn out their bird seed cake. It can be hung up for birds to find.

Use this as an opportunity to talk to children about seeds that they may eat, e.g. breakfast cereals, breads, etc. Encourage them to notice that people have different preferences and that these differences are interesting.

Health and safety
♦ Lard melts very quickly, especially in a microwave. You may wish to melt the lard away from the children to avoid accidents.
♦ Supervise this activity carefully to ensure that children do not eat any of the bird seed or dried items.
♦ Do not include any nuts or products containing traces of nuts, if you are working with a child with a nut allergy.
♦ Check with parents that they have no objection to the use of lard, as it is an animal fat.

Extending and varying children's learning
♦ Provide books about different types of birds, or stories that have a bird as a central theme.
♦ Follow this activity with children making their own muesli.
♦ Bring in wheat germ and show children how when it is ground it makes flour.
♦ Read the nursery rhyme 'Birds of the air' (*Collins Book of Nursery Rhymes*).

2 Role-play area: Garden centre

Do you know where we can buy plants? A garden centre sells plants, seeds, sheds, and everything for a garden.

Specific resources
♦ plant pots
♦ bags
♦ empty seed packets
♦ bottles
♦ catalogues and pictures of plants
♦ other available items including tools
♦ play money
♦ calculator
♦ jars
♦ shop till
♦ bags of sand, gravel and soil

Key learning intentions
This activity helps children use language for communication and use numbers as labels by using play money.

Links to Foundation Stage curriculum

Area of learning	Aspects of learning	Curriculum guidance page
Personal, social and emotional development	Disposition and attitudes Self-confidence and self-esteem Making relationships Behaviour and self-control Self-care	32 34 36 38 40
Communication, language and literacy	Language for communication Language for thinking Writing	48, 50, 52, 54 56–8 64
Mathematical development	Numbers as labels and for counting Calculating Shape, space and measures	74 76 78–80
Knowledge and understanding of the world	Designing and making skills Information and communication technology Sense of time Sense of place	90 92 94 96
Physical development	Sense of space Using tools and materials	104 114
Creative development	Exploring media and materials Imagination Responding to experiences, and expressing and communicating ideas	120 124 126

Ideas for organising the activity

The role-play area is an excellent way of helping children to use language and to make relationships. Begin by making sure that children understand what a garden centre does. If children have no experience of garden centres, you may wish to visit one. The starting point for an effective role-play area is to present materials, but also to encourage children to make items for the area themselves. They can plant seeds, put soil into bags, make labels for prices and arrange items on shelves.

Show children how a calculator works to encourage them to talk about numbers and to learn how to use this piece of ICT equipment.

Extending and varying children's learning

◆ Children can hold a real plant sale.
◆ Encourage children to 'play' write orders down.
◆ Ask children to organise items by size in the shop.
◆ Children can decorate plant pots and make paper flowers.

3 Beans in the egg boxes

Let's play a game with the beans and the egg boxes.

Specific resources

◆ egg boxes   ◆ beans

Key learning intentions
This activity will help children to one-to-one match, to use numbers to count with and also to count.

Links to Foundation Stage curriculum		
Area of learning	**Aspects of learning**	**Curriculum guidance page**
Personal, social and emotional development	Disposition and attitudes Behaviour and self-control	32 38
Communication, language and literacy	Language for communication Language for thinking	48, 50, 52, 54 56–8
Mathematical development	Numbers as labels and for counting Calculating Shape, space and measures	74 76 78–80
Physical development	Movement Using tools and materials	106, 108 114
Creative development	Exploring media and materials	120

Ideas for organising the activity

This activity works well with two or three children at a time, although the same resources should be put out on another table so that they can leave you and then carry on playing if they choose.

Begin by letting the children put beans in and out of the egg boxes. Ask them if they can put one bean in each section. Do they know how many beans there are? With older children, you could ask them to put two beans in each section so that they count in pairs. Now play a game where the children cover their eyes and you take some beans out. Do they know how many beans are left? How many have been taken out? They can look in the palm of your hand to see if they are right. Repeat the game with children taking it in turns to take beans out of the egg box and the others guessing or counting how many they have in their hand.

Use this activity to encourage children to talk about their homes – do they have any plants indoors? Do they ever plant seeds or beans?

Extending and varying children's learning
◆ Cut the egg box into a strip of three for younger children.
◆ Play a game where children roll the dice and put in the number of beans that are shown on the dice.
◆ Use this as a way of practising number bonds to six with older reception children.
◆ Put out a tray of beans and a spoon and ask children if they can spoon in one bean to each section.
◆ Use a pair of tweezers and ask children if they can take out the number of beans shown on the dice with the tweezers.

4 Hunt the beans and seeds

A few days ago, the bean fairy planted some beans in the outdoor area. Let's look and see if we can find anything that is beginning to grow.

Specific resources
◆ sticks or straws   ◆ beans   ◆ pencils and paper

Key learning intentions
This activity helps children to observe their outdoor area closely and note changes and differences.

Links to Foundation Stage curriculum

Area of learning	Aspects of learning	Curriculum guidance page
Personal, social and emotional development	Disposition and attitudes Behaviour and self-control Self-care Sense of community	32 38 40 42
Communication, language and literacy	Language for communication Language for thinking Reading Writing	48, 50, 52, 54 56–8 62 64
Mathematical development	Numbers as labels and for counting Shape, space and measures	74 78–80

Knowledge and understanding of the world	Exploration and investigation Sense of time Sense of place	86, 88 94 96
Physical development	Sense of space Movement Using tools and materials	104 106, 108 114
Creative development	Exploring media and materials Responding to experiences, and expressing and communicating ideas	120 126

Ideas for organising the activity

This activity needs preparing in advance. Plant twenty or so beans in pots outdoors or in borders, if these are available. Make sure that they will be easily seen when they begin to sprout.

Once they are beginning to push through the soil, take small groups of children out to hunt for them. You can weave a story if you wish about a bean fairy who was passing by and who dropped the beans for the children to find. This activity also links to *Jack and the Beanstalk*! Children can make maps and make markers to show where all the beans are hidden.

Extending and varying children's learning

◆ Watch the beans as they grow – were some actually weeds?
◆ Measure the beans.
◆ Make maps of other features in the outdoor area.
◆ Give other seeds for children to plant and recreate the bean fairy.
◆ Take photographs as the beans grow – children can adopt a bean!

5 Find the beans hidden in the rice

Teddy has been playing tricks on us – he has hidden some beans amongst the coloured rice! He wants us to see if we can find them and take them out.

Specific resources

◆ coloured rice
◆ tweezers
◆ chopsticks

◆ beans
◆ spoons
◆ bowls

Key learning intentions
This activity develops children's fine motor skills and their use of tools.

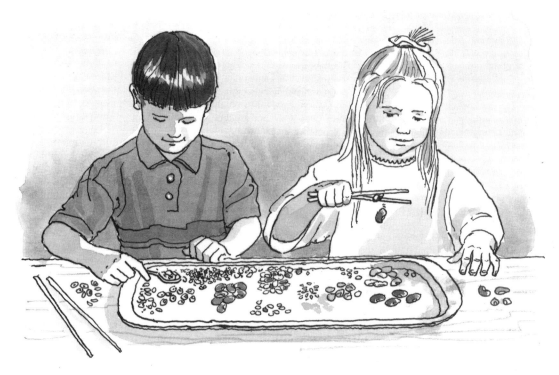

This activity can be made simpler by letting them take the beans out with their hands

Links to Foundation Stage curriculum		
Area of learning	**Aspects of learning**	**Curriculum guidance page**
Personal, social and emotional development	Disposition and attitudes Making relationships Self-care Sense of community	32 36 40 42
Communication, language and literacy	Language for communication Language for thinking Handwriting	48, 50, 52, 54 56–8 66
Mathematical development	Numbers as labels and for counting Calculating Shape, space and measures	74 76 78–80
Knowledge and understanding of the world	Exploration and investigation	86, 88
Physical development	Movement Using tools and materials	106, 108 114
Creative development	Exploring media and materials Imagination	120 124

Ideas for organising the activity

Begin by preparing the rice – simply put some rice into a carrier bag, add a few drops of food colouring and shake. Once the rice has taken on the colour, spread it out on a baking sheet and put it either in a warm place or an oven so that it can dry.

This activity works well with pairs of children. Put the rice into a tray and add in some beans. Using teddy as a stooge, tell the children that teddy has been playing tricks. He wants to see if we can get the beans out without using our hands – can we use tweezers, spoons or even chopsticks to pick up the beans! As the beans are being taken out, children can count how many beans teddy dropped in! This activity can be made simpler by letting them take the beans out with their hands.

Extending and varying children's learning

- Teddy may play other tricks – smaller seeds can be put into the rice tray.
- Children can write to teddy to tell him that they can take the seeds out!
- Children can hide other things in the rice tray – to see if we can take them out!
- Can children find the beans using their hands, but not looking?

6 Paper plate flowers

Would you like to make your own flower to go in a pot?

Specific resources

- pebbles
- glue
- scissors
- lace
- ribbons
- collage materials
- paper plates – different sizes
- plastic plant pots – various sizes
- a good selection of paper, e.g. tissue paper, coloured paper, gummed paper
- wooden green sticks (usually from garden centres) or straws

---

Key learning intentions

This activity is designed for children to use a range of materials and to enjoy creating their own flowers. These can be used later as part of a display.

Links to Foundation Stage curriculum

Area of learning	Aspects of learning	Curriculum guidance page
Personal, social and emotional development	Disposition and attitudes Behaviour and self-control Self-care	32 38 40
Communication, language and literacy	Language for communication Language for thinking Reading Writing Handwriting	48, 50, 52, 54 56–8 62 64 66

▽

Mathematical development	Numbers as labels and for counting	74
	Calculating	76
	Shape, space and measures	78–80
Knowledge and understanding of the world	Exploration and investigation	86, 88
	Designing and making skills	90
Physical development	Movement	106, 108
	Using tools and materials	114
Creative development	Exploring media and materials	120
	Music	122
	Imagination	124
	Responding to experiences, and expressing and communicating ideas	126

Ideas for organising the activity

This activity works well with small groups of children or pairs. Show children the paper plate, green stick and materials that can be collaged to form a flower. Ask them if they can see how to make a flower using the paper plate as a base for putting petals on.

The aim of this activity is to encourage children to problem solve as well as be creative. While you may have to help them to cut shapes or find ways of sticking, it is important that they keep control and follow their own ideas – this may mean not producing a prototype you have made in advance, as the danger is that this will influence their decisions. The flowers can be put into pots filled with pebbles or other materials, or used for a display. Encourage children to find ways of marking their names on their work, e.g. they may add a label with their name or tell you what makes their work stand out.

Extending and varying children's learning

- Ask the children if they would like to put a photograph of someone they care for in the centre of their flower.
- Bring in 'daisy' shaped flowers for children to dissect – model the vocabulary of flowers, e.g. stem, stamen, leaves.
- Bring in fresh flowers for children to arrange into florist's oasis – this needs to be soaked overnight to keep the flowers fresh.
- Look at ways in which flowers are used to celebrate occasions, e.g. weddings, Mother's day.
- Repeat this activity, but group flowers, e.g. one flower in a pot, two flowers in a pot, to help children use numbers as labels and for counting.

Theme 16 Shells

Shells are interesting for children as they come in unusual shapes. Children are often fascinated by their colours and some children have seen shells on beaches. Shells can be used as a starting point to talk about the sea and things that are found in the sea.

Inside the box on each area of learning below is a range of ideas for activities and stories on the theme of shells. You will find on the following pages a ready-made activity plan for the first idea listed in each box. In addition, all the stories mentioned are listed in the Booklist on pages 250–252.

Ideas to suggest to parents
◆ Show their child any of your holiday photos – especially if taken at the seaside.
◆ Point out any shells or shell shapes that they see, e.g. soaps, designs on towels.
◆ Look out for snails in parks, gardens or other outdoor spaces.

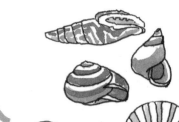

Personal, social and emotional development
◆ *Activity plan: Teddy's seaside holiday (p. 202)*
◆ Using shells to decorate an area of the garden or a plant tub.
◆ Making a frame with shells for a special photograph.
◆ In pairs, look at these shells – do you have the same favourites?

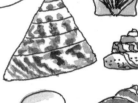
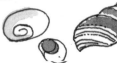

Communication, language and literacy
◆ *Activity plan: Mark making in the sand with shells (p. 203)*
◆ Stories:
    ◆ *The Hare and the Tortoise*
    ◆ *Meg at Sea*
    ◆ *Smelly Jelly, Smelly Fish*
    ◆ *Snail Trail*
    ◆ *Turtle Bay*
    ◆ *Who Are You in the Sea?*
◆ Nursery rhyme: 'Mary, Mary, quite contrary, how does your garden grow?'
◆ Role-play area: Souvenir and gift shop.
◆ Hard and soft – feely bag game.
◆ I am describing a shell – can you work out which one?
◆ Kim's game: Which shell is missing?

Creative development

- *Activity plan: Can you make a box for teddy's favourite shell? (p. 208)*
- Dancing and making spirals and twists like the conch shells.
- Making shell shakers.
- Make shell people – stick faces onto shells.
- Collages with various materials including shells.
- Observational drawing and painting of shells.

Physical development

- *Activity plan: Follow the line with the shell (p. 207)*
- Can you find the shell hidden in the sand tray?
- Parachute games – cockles, whelks and mussels (see p. 185).
- Shell prints in the dough.
- Shell and spoon obstacle races.
- Which of these shells can you make roll?
- Hunt the shells that are hidden outside.
- Scoop water with flat shells.

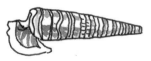

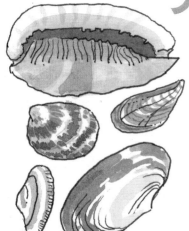

Knowledge and understanding of the world

- *Activity plan: Pebbles and shells (p. 206)*
- Shells in the water tray – can you make any shells float?
- Look at these shells with the magnifying glass – can you see the ridges on the shells?
- Can you use the remote-controlled car to go in and out of an obstacle course with shells?
- Let's look outside – can we see any snails? – Snails have shells.
- Look at this snail on the window outside – can you see how it moves?

Mathematical development

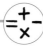

- *Activity plan: How much water does this shell hold? (p. 204)*
- Count shells.
- How many shells will fit into this little box?
- How many shells in the feely bag – one, two, three or more?
- Sort shells into sizes.
- Which is the best size of box for this shell?

Activity plans for the theme 'shells'

I Teddy's seaside holiday

Teddy has brought his story bag with him. What has he got to show us today? Where has he been? What do you think he has been doing?

Specific resources

- teddy
- T-shirt
- fabric bag or box
- water wings
- shells
- postcard to the children from teddy
- sun cream

Key learning intentions

This activity should help children to talk about doing things that they enjoy at home.
It should also help them to think about safety.

Links to Foundation Stage curriculum

Area of learning	Aspects of learning	Curriculum guidance page
Personal, social and emotional development	Disposition and attitudes Self-confidence and self-esteem Making relationships Behaviour and self-control Self-care Sense of community	32 34 36 38 40 42
Communication, language and literacy	Language for communication Language for thinking Linking sounds with letters Reading	48, 50, 52, 54 56–8 60 62
Mathematical development	Numbers as labels and for counting	74
Knowledge and understanding of the world	Exploration and investigation Sense of time Sense of place	86, 88 94 96
Physical development	Sense of space Health and bodily awareness	104 110
Creative development	Exploring media and materials Imagination Responding to experiences, and expressing and communicating ideas	120 124 126

Ideas for organising the activity

This activity is designed for small groups of children so that they can freely pass comments. Ask them if they can guess what teddy might have in his bag. Take out the objects one by one. How many objects has he got in his bag? Pass them around so that children can feel and talk about them. Do any of the objects have an 's' sound? What do they think teddy has been doing?

Tell them that teddy has been away with his family. Have they ever gone on holiday or been away with their families? Tell them that teddy had gone to the seaside and that it was very hot. Ask the children if they can guess why he needed sun cream. Use the water wings to talk about safety in the water. The children can ask teddy if he was sensible in the water – what did he do? Use this type of activity as a way of encouraging children to ask teddy other questions.

Finally, discover the postcard that teddy has written to the children. Read it to the children and pass it around so that they can see it.

Extending and varying children's learning

◆ Teddy has brought back some postcards – could the children write on them?
◆ Leave the story bag out (remove the sun cream) so that the children can recreate the story.
◆ Put out sequencing cards – teddy packing the case, teddy going in the car, teddy playing on the beach – can the children put them in the correct order?

2 Mark making in the sand with shells

Look at how you can draw in the sand with shells and make shapes.

Specific resources

◆ damp sand   ◆ shells   ◆ shallow trays of sand (optional)

Key learning intentions
This activity should encourage children to make large marks or to 'write' in the sand. It will encourage children's fine manipulative skills as well as hand-eye co-ordination.

Links to Foundation Stage curriculum		
Area of learning	**Aspects of learning**	**Curriculum guidance page**
Personal, social and emotional development	Disposition and attitudes Self-confidence and self-esteem Self-care	32 34 40
Communication, language and literacy	Language for communication Language for thinking Handwriting	48, 50, 52, 54 56–8 66
Mathematical development	Shape, space and measures	78–80
Knowledge and understanding of the world	Exploration and investigation Designing and making skills	86, 88 90
Physical development	Movement Using tools and materials	106, 108 114
Creative development	Exploring media and materials	120

Ideas for organising the activity

Put damp sand out either in the sand tray or in shallow trays (new cat litter trays are ideal for this!) Put out a range of shells including some with pointed ends.

Ask children if they would like to write 'magic' messages in the sand. Show them how they can 'rub out' the message by simply sweeping over the sand with their hand or a flat shell. Encourage them to make large marks so that they develop fluent movements, which are essential for handwriting. Children who are interested in letter shapes will benefit from having letters and name cards nearby so that they can reproduce letters.

Health and safety
As with any activity involving sand, good supervision is required to prevent sand being thrown about.

Extending and varying children's learning
- Children can write notes on paper to hide in the sand.
- Children can hide notes under or in the shells and then put them into the sand.
- Children can draw pictures in the sand and decorate them with shells.
- Ask children to take it in turns to make prints in the sand with a shell. The other children have to work out which shell was used to make the print.

3 How much water does this shell hold?

Look at all these shells in the water tray. Which shell do you think will hold the most water?

Specific resources
- a range of shells including 'flat' shells such as mussels, as well as spiral shells
- clear beakers to measure water
- egg cups

Key learning intentions
This activity will help children to measure and to count. They will also learn the skills of observation and exploration.

Links to Foundation Stage curriculum		
Area of learning	**Aspects of learning**	**Curriculum guidance page**
Personal, social and emotional development	Disposition and attitudes Self-confidence and self-esteem Behaviour and self-control Self-care	32 34 38 40
Communication, language and literacy	Language for communication Language for thinking	48, 50, 52, 54 56–8

▽

Mathematical development	Numbers as labels and for counting Calculating Shape, space and measures	74 76 78–80
Knowledge and understanding of the world	Exploration and investigation	86, 88
Physical development	Movement Using equipment Using tools and materials	106, 108 112 114
Creative development	Exploring media and materials	120

Ideas for organising the activity

Put a selection of shells in the water tray for children to enjoy playing with. Ask individuals or pairs which shell they think will hold the most water. Encourage them to think about how they could measure the amount of water a shell could hold.

Let them experiment with different shells. Which shell holds the most? You could also ask them to work out how many 'shellfuls' of water would be needed to fill an egg cup.

Extending and varying children's learning

◆ Compare the capacity of a shell to that of a sponge.
◆ Encourage children to match the following labels to the shells: 'most' 'least'.
◆ Ask the children to consider if the heavier shells will hold more?
◆ Produce an interest table that shows which shells hold the most water.

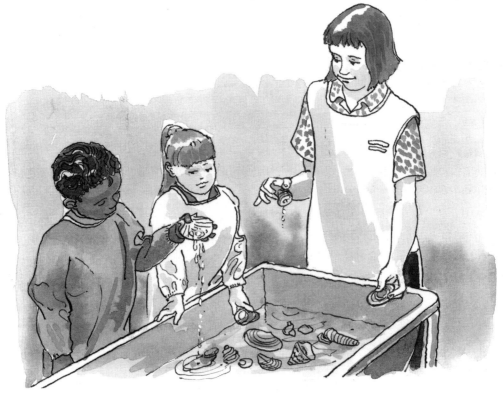

Which shell holds the most?

4 Pebbles and shells

Here are some small pebbles and here are some shells. What are the differences between them?

Specific resources

◆ tray of shells and pebbles ◆ small boxes ◆ access to water ◆ scales

---

Key learning intentions

This activity is designed to help children to explore materials and to notice similarities and differences.

Links to Foundation Stage curriculum

Area of learning	Aspects of learning	Curriculum guidance page
Personal, social and emotional development	Disposition and attitudes Behaviour and self-control Self-care	32 38 40
Communication, language and literacy	Language for communication Language for thinking	48, 50, 52, 54 56–8
Mathematical development	Numbers as labels and for counting Calculating Shape, space and measures	74 76 78–80
Knowledge and understanding of the world	Exploration and investigation	86, 88
Physical development	Using equipment Using tools and materials	112 114
Creative development	Exploring media and materials Responding to experiences, and expressing and communicating ideas	120 126

Ideas for organising the activity

This activity works well with pairs and small groups of children. Put out a tray of shells and pebbles (with a small group, provide several trays so that children can be active). Ask the children if they can tell you what is in the tray – some children may use the word stones, but will need to hear the word 'pebble' modelled. Use this as an opportunity to ask them if they have seen shells before and where they have seen them.

You may also see if the children know the names of any of the shells. Ask them if they can sort out the shells from the pebbles. What makes them different? What can pebbles do that shells cannot? Do pebbles float or sink? Can pebbles roll? Which is heavier – a shell or a pebble that you can put in the palm of your hand? Ask the children to count how many pebbles they have found amongst the shells.

Extending and varying children's learning

◆ Ask the children to choose their favourite shell or pebble. Why do they like it?
◆ Ask the children to order the shells and pebbles according to size.
◆ How many shells are needed to balance these three pebbles?
◆ Can you make a straight line/circle using the shells?

5 Follow the line with the shell

Look at this shell. If you put your finger on it gently, you can make it move. Can you now follow the line with the shell?

Specific resources

◆ small shells that are easy to move along a flat surface with the tip of a finger

> **Key learning intentions**
> This activity is to help children's hand-eye co-ordination and develop fluid movements in their wrists.

Links to Foundation Stage curriculum		
Area of learning	**Aspects of learning**	**Curriculum guidance page**
Personal, social and emotional development	Disposition and attitudes Self-confidence and self-esteem	32 34
Communication, language and literacy	Language for communication Language for thinking Handwriting	48, 50, 52, 54 56–8 66
Mathematical development	Numbers as labels and for counting	74
Knowledge and understanding of the world	Exploration and investigation	86, 88
Physical development	Movement Using equipment	106, 108 112
Creative development	Exploring media and materials Imagination	120 124

Ideas for organising the activity

This activity works well with pairs or individual children. Put out a selection of small shells. Ask the children if they can choose one shell and show them how you can move it with the tip of the index finger. Encourage them – if they press too hard, the shell will not move easily.

Once the children are able to move the shell, draw a line on a piece of paper. Ask if they would like to take their shell for a walk along the line – this may need demonstrating! Do not focus on accuracy, the main purpose of this activity is to encourage their overall hand development.

Extending and varying children's learning
- Ask children if they would like to draw their own line to follow.
- Draw two parallel lines that curve and twist – can children keep their shell in the middle of the road?
- Repeat this activity in the sand pit with dry sand.
- Encourage children to make specific movements, e.g. circular movements, waves and vertical movements.
- Encourage children to make up their own story, e.g. what is happening as the shell is going for a walk?

6 Can you make a box for teddy's favourite shell?

Which shell do you like? Have you a favourite? Teddy has a favourite shell that he wants to take home. Can you make a special box or bag for it?

Specific resources
- paper
- crayons
- card
- scissors
- stapler
- sticky tape
- small boxes

Key learning intentions

This activity should help children to explore a range of materials, use tools and problem solve.

Links to Foundation Stage curriculum

Area of learning	Aspects of learning	Curriculum guidance page
Personal, social and emotional development	Disposition and attitudes Self-confidence and self-esteem Making relationships Behaviour and self-control Self-care	32 34 36 38 40
Communication, language and literacy	Language for communication Language for thinking	48, 50, 52, 54 56–8
Mathematical development	Calculating Shape, space and measures	76 78–80
Knowledge and understanding of the world	Exploration and investigation Designing and making skills	86, 88 90
Physical development	Movement Using equipment Using tools and materials	106, 108 112 114
Creative development	Exploring media and materials Imagination Responding to experiences, and expressing and communicating ideas	120 124 126

Ideas for organising the activity

This activity can be carried out with small groups of children or pairs. Put out a range of shells for children to hold and touch. Using teddy as a stooge, ask them which shell they think teddy might like best. Encourage them to say why they have chosen the shell.

Say that teddy would like to take the shell home and could they make something for teddy to keep it in. Show them the resources available – if they are unfamiliar with using a stapler, show them how to use it. This activity should be a creative one, with teddy being pleased with anything that is produced! Encourage the children to 'write' a note so that teddy will remember what is in his box or bag!

Extending and varying children's learning

◆ Children can decorate boxes with shells.
◆ Teddy can send a thank-you letter to the children.
◆ Find out from children if they have 'precious' things at home.

Theme 17 Spoons

Spoons are an everyday feature of most children's lives. This theme is a good starting point to talk about the differences in people's diets and ways of eating. It can also develop into looking at kitchens and cooking.

Inside the box on each area of learning below is a range of ideas for activities and stories on the theme of spoons. You will find on the following pages a ready-made activity plan for the first idea listed in each box. In addition, all the stories mentioned are listed in the Booklist on pages 250–252.

Ideas to suggest to parents

◆ Point out different types of spoons in their home, e.g. ladle, teaspoon, tablespoon, baby spoon.

◆ Talk to their child about the uses of different types of spoon.

◆ Try a simple cooking activity with their child involving stirring and mixing.

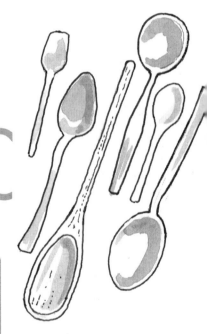

Personal, social and emotional development

◆ *Activity plan: Try a spoonful of this (p. 212)*

◆ Washing and drying cutlery and plates with an adult.

◆ Laying out a place setting.

◆ Tidying up the cutlery drawer – knives, forks and spoons.

◆ Display: Photographs of important meals in children's lives.

Communication, language and literacy

◆ *Activity plan: Role-play area: Our dining area (p. 213)*

◆ Stories:
  ◆ *Honey Biscuits*
  ◆ *The Tiger Who Came to Tea*

◆ Rhyme: 'Here's the lady's knives and forks' (*Round and Round the Garden*)

◆ Do you know the name of these spoons?

◆ Feely bag: Can you guess what type of spoon you are feeling?

◆ Song: 'Hey diddle, diddle . . .'

◆ Mark making – spoons in the sand.

◆ Kim's game: Spoons, knives, chopsticks, forks, bowls – what has disappeared?

◆ Story bag (apron, wooden spoon, recipe book): What has teddy been doing?

Creative development

- Activity plan: *Mixing paints (p. 218)*
- What sounds can you make with these spoons?
- Listen to the spoons being passed around the circle – who has them now?
- Role-play area: Kitchen shop.

Physical development

- *Activity plan: Spoon races (p. 217)*
- Cornflour and water – mix and play with spoons.
- Spoons of different sizes with dough.
- Spoons and plastic bottles in the sand and water tray.
- Spoons, knives and forks in the sand tray.
- Scoops and spoons with coloured rice.

Knowledge and understanding of the world

- *Activity plan: Stirring – can you make stretchy dough? (p. 215)*
- Look at these different spoons – can you find those made from wood?
- Guess which of these spoons will float.
- Do you use any of these at meal times in your home – chopsticks, knives, forks, spoons, finger bowls, napkins?
- Sort spoons – size, colour, length.
- Let's make a drink – shall we mix some different fruit juices together?

Mathematical development

- *Activity plan: Guess which spoon! (p. 214)*
- Which spoon would be the best to use to empty this tall, thin container?
- Throw the dice and put in the number of spoonfuls of water into your beaker – when the beaker is full you have won.
- Which holds the most – a heaped or a level spoon?

Activity plans for the theme 'spoons'

1 Try a spoonful of this

Here are some different foods for you to taste. Take a spoonful – what do you think?

Specific resources

- plastic or metal teaspoon
- plastic plates
- paper napkins
- a selection of sweet and savoury foods – choice depends on cost and also dietary needs of children in your setting

---

Key learning intentions

This activity helps children to talk about foods they like and dislike and to realise that people have different taste preferences.

Links to Foundation Stage curriculum

Area of learning	Aspects of learning	Curriculum guidance page
Personal, social and emotional development	Disposition and attitudes Self-confidence and self-esteem Making relationships Behaviour and self-control	32 34 36 38
Communication, language and literacy	Language for communication Language for thinking Reading	48, 50, 52, 54 56–8 62
Knowledge and understanding of the world	Exploration and investigation	86, 88
Physical development	Using tools and materials	114
Creative development	Imagination	124

Ideas for organising the activity

This activity works well with groups of up to five children. Begin by putting out a selection of foods that children may not recognise with a serving spoon. Ask each child to choose a spoon and a plate. They should help themselves to a selection of foods.

Encourage children to guess whether it will be savoury or sweet. Can they guess from the colour? Ask children to taste using the spoons. Are there some flavours that they prefer? Encourage children to notice that others in the group may not have the same preference. Use this activity to talk about the way in which we all have different likes and dislikes.

Health and safety

As with any activity involving food, it is essential to check beforehand that any food offered will meet with children's dietary needs.

Extending and varying children's learning

◆ Ask children to choose a favourite food.
◆ Children can draw pictures or cut out pictures of their favourite foods.
◆ Read the story *Oliver's Vegetables* about a child who only likes certain foods.
◆ Take photographs of children as they are doing this activity – use for a display!

2 Role-play area: Our dining area

Look at the home area – today we have a kitchen and a table to eat on.

Specific resources

◆ plastic plates	◆ bowls	◆ cups
◆ plastic cutlery	◆ play dough	◆ dry rice
◆ pasta	◆ rolling pins	◆ range of cookery books

◆ cooking equipment found in the homes of children you are working with

---

Key learning intentions

This activity will help children use language relating to cooking and eating. It will also develop children's imagination and fine motor skills.

Links to Foundation Stage curriculum

Area of learning	Aspects of learning	Curriculum guidance page
Personal, social and emotional development	Disposition and attitudes Self-confidence and self-esteem Making relationships Behaviour and self-control Sense of community	32 34 36 38 42
Communication, language and literacy	Language for communication Language for thinking Reading	48, 50, 52, 54 56–8 62
Mathematical development	Numbers as labels and for counting Calculating Shape, space and measures	74 76 78-80
Knowledge and understanding of the world	Sense of place Cultures and beliefs	96 98
Physical development	Movement Using equipment Using tools and materials	106, 108 112 114
Creative development	Exploring media and materials Imagination	120 124

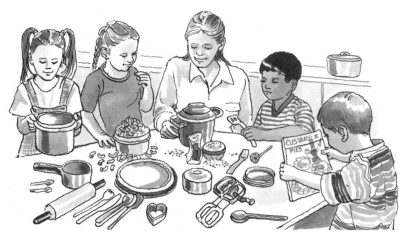

Spend time playing alongside children to model language

Ideas for organising the activity

This is an ideal way of helping children to learn the language connected to eating and cooking. Make sure props reflect children's home backgrounds by asking parents to bring in any spare utensils, cookery books, etc. Encourage children to play by showing them cookery books and asking them if they would like to pretend to cook. Provide materials such as play dough, dried rice, pasta, etc. to make the play as realistic as possible. Spend some time playing alongside children to model language, especially where they have a different home language to the one used in the setting.

Extending and varying children's learning

- Children can play 'washing up'.
- Introduce cuddly toys and dolls for children to feed and look after.
- Take pictures of children in the role-play area.
- Provide pens, paper, glue and pictures of food so that children can make their own cookery books and menus.
- Develop the theme further by adding in shopping lists, shopping baskets so that children 'buy' food.

3 Guess which spoon!

There are three spoons here. Guess which of these spoons held this amount of sand?

Specific resources

- water
- sand
- containers
- several spoons, e.g. teaspoon, tablespoon, ladle or serving spoon

> **Key learning intentions**
> This activity should help children to compare two groups as well as learn practically about capacity.

Links to Foundation Stage curriculum		
Area of learning	**Aspects of learning**	**Curriculum guidance page**
Personal, social and emotional development	Disposition and attitudes Behaviour and self-control	32 38
Communication, language and literacy	Language for communication Language for thinking	48, 50, 52, 54 56–8
Mathematical development	Numbers as labels and for counting Calculating Shape, space and measures	74 76 78–80
Physical development	Sense of space Movement Using equipment	104 106, 108 112

Ideas for organising the activity

This activity works best with individual children or pairs. Begin by showing children the spoons that you have chosen. If they are very young or need support in their mathematics, put out only two or three spoons. Encourage them to play with them in the sand or water – whichever material you are working with first. Tell them that they are going to play a game.

Take a spoonful of sand and put it into a beaker or onto a tray so that the children can see it easily. Ask them if they can guess which spoon you used. Play the game again, but this time they can put out the spoonful and you must guess! Model language of quantity to children by using words such as 'most' 'least', 'small', 'large', etc. Once they have begun to be accurate in their guessing, use one spoon and ask them to guess the number of spoonfuls you have put out – one or two! Again, they can play this game on you.

Extending and varying children's learning

◆ Repeat this game using a variety of different media, e.g. cooked rice, buttons, water.
◆ Encourage older children to play this game in pairs with each other.
◆ Ask children to 'match' by guessing the spoon and then putting a spoonful alongside yours.

4 Stirring – can you make stretchy dough?

Feel this dough – would you like to make your own?

Specific resources

◆ self-raising flour
◆ food colouring

◆ bowls
◆ selection of spoons

◆ water
◆ small jugs

Key learning intentions
This activity is designed for children to notice changes in materials and to develop their fine motor skills.

Links to Foundation Stage curriculum

Area of learning	Aspects of learning	Curriculum guidance page
Personal, social and emotional development	Disposition and attitudes Self-confidence and self-esteem Sense of community	32 34 42
Communication, language and literacy	Language for communication Language for thinking	48, 50, 52, 54 56–8
Mathematical development	Numbers as labels and for counting Calculating Shape, space and measures	74 76 78–80
Knowledge and understanding of the world	Exploration and investigation Designing and making skills Sense of time	86, 88 90 94
Physical development	Using equipment Using tools and materials	112 114
Creative development	Imagination	124

Ideas for organising the activity

This activity works well with pairs of children or small groups. Begin by showing children some stretchy dough that has been made with coloured water and self-raising flour. Ask them if they would like to make their own dough to play with.

Let every child choose a bowl, a jug and a spoon. Ask them to get some water by pouring water from a bottle into their jug. Give them a choice of food colouring and see if they can put a few drops into their water. Using a larger spoon, ask them to take some self-raising flour and put it into their bowl. They can gradually pour water and stir the mixture. Talk to them about the texture and the feel of their emerging dough. Encourage them to problem solve – do they need to add more water or more flour to their mixture? Model the language of cooking, e.g. 'knead', 'roll', 'stir', 'sticky', and encourage them to explore its properties – what has happened to the flour?

Health and safety
As with any activity involving food, check that children do not have any allergies, e.g. wheat allergies.

Stretchy dough does not contain salt and therefore must be thrown away at the end of the session.

This activity will need supervising and children should be discouraged from eating the dough.

Extending and varying children's learning

◆ Provide children with a different type of dough – what differences do they notice?
◆ Put out spoons, knives and scissors with the dough so that they can enjoy cutting and shaping it.
◆ Play mathematical games such as 'roll a dice' – the children split their dough into the number of pieces shown on the dice.
◆ Children repeat making dough using a variety of flours, e.g. wholemeal, granary.
◆ Children 'write' down or draw the recipe for stretchy dough.

5 Spoon races

Look at these objects. Can you choose the best spoon to transport them along this chalk line?

Specific resources

◆ a range of small objects of different sizes, e.g. buttons, beanbags, balls, marbles
◆ range of spoons   ◆ chalk

Key learning intentions

This activity is designed to help children's fine and locomotive skills. It also provides an opportunity to problem solve.

Links to Foundation Stage curriculum

Area of learning	Aspects of learning	Curriculum guidance page
Personal, social and emotional development	Disposition and attitudes Making relationships Behaviour and self-control	32 36 38
Knowledge and understanding of the world	Designing and making skills	90
Physical development	Sense of space Movement Using tools and development	104 106, 108 114
Communication, language and literacy	Language for communication Language for thinking Writing	48, 50, 52, 54 56–8 64
Creative development	Imagination Responding to experiences, and expressing and communicating ideas	124 126

Ideas for organising the activity

This activity works well with pairs or small groups. Show children the collection of objects and the spoons. Ask them if they can choose an object to put in their spoon. Can they walk without it falling off?

If children are enjoying trying this, draw a chalk line 'road' and see if they can follow the road. Are there any spoons that are better than others for carrying objects? Is it easier to carry something on a large or a small spoon? Draw other roads – is it easier to walk on a straight line or a curvy one?

Use this activity to model language, especially for describing movements and position.

Extending and varying children's learning

◆ Children can draw chalk lines and make their own games.
◆ Encourage children to choose other items to transport the objects, e.g. boxes, trays.
◆ Repeat this activity but devise an obstacle course.

6 Mixing paints

Come and look at these lovely paints. Shall we see how many colours we can make?

Specific resources

◆ tablespoons
◆ teaspoons
◆ plastic beakers or paint pots
◆ large sheets of paper or lining paper
◆ trays
◆ sponges
◆ rollers
◆ masking tape
◆ plastic sheeting
◆ ready-mixed paint – red, yellow, blue and white
◆ a range of paintbrushes including some large ones

Key learning intentions
This activity will help children to explore colour whilst developing fine and gross motor skills to make marks.

Links to Foundation Stage curriculum

Area of learning	Aspects of learning	Curriculum guidance page
Personal, social and emotional development	Disposition and attitudes	32
Communication, language and literacy	Language for communication Language for thinking	48, 50, 52, 54 56–8
Mathematical development	Shape, space and measures	78–80
Knowledge and understanding of the world	Designing and making skills Information and communication technology	90 92
Physical development	Using tools and materials	114
Creative development	Exploring media and materials Responding to experiences, and expressing and communicating ideas	120 126

Ideas for organising the activity

This activity works well with pairs or individuals. Put the primary colours into beakers or pots and a tablespoon in each beaker or pot. Place sheets of plastic, held in place with masking tape, on a wall so that children will be able to make large marks.

Give each child a tray and ask them to use the tablespoons to put a spoonful of each colour onto the tray. Ask them to take a teaspoon and take a little bit of one colour and slowly mix it with another – you may need to demonstrate on your own tray. Once they can see a new colour ask them to put a little of it onto the paper. Encourage them to use whatever tool they wish, e.g. sponge, paintbrush, cloth, etc.

Ask them to guess how many colours they might find! Encourage them to name the colours or to invent words for their new colours based on their experiences, e.g. sky blue, my bedroom red! Once they have finished exploring the colours, encourage them to clean their own trays, by putting it under a tap and wiping it. This will help develop their self-esteem and self-help skills.

Extending and varying children's learning

◆ Encourage children to learn about shades of colour by mixing a colour with white paint.
◆ Use paint cards to see if children can match any of their colours to the cards.
◆ Use the painting wall – encourage children to paint large pictures.

Theme 18 Teddy bears

Most children have a teddy bear at home or can recognise a teddy bear. This theme is particularly good for encouraging children to talk about their feelings and lends itself to plenty of language activities.

Inside the box on each area of learning below is a range of ideas for activities and stories on the theme of teddy bears. You will find on the following pages a ready-made activity plan for the first idea listed in each box. In addition, all the stories mentioned are listed in the Booklist on pages 250–252.

Ideas to suggest to parents
◆ Point out teddy bears to their child, e.g. on clothes, in books, in shops.
◆ Read a book about a bear, perhaps one of the examples below.
◆ Encourage their child to make something for their teddy bear or favourite cuddly toy.

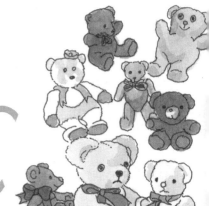

Personal, social and emotional development
◆ *Activity plan: This is the Bear and the Scary Night* (p. 222)
◆ Display: 'These are things that help me to get to sleep.'
◆ Teddy is feeling sad – can we help him to feel better?
◆ Guess which of these are teddy's favourite toys.
◆ Tell teddy about your family.
◆ Show teddy how you can tidy up.

Communication, language and literacy
◆ *Activity plan: Guess what teddy can do* (p. 223)
◆ Hunt the hidden teddies – can you tell teddy where his friends are hiding?
◆ Kim's game: Which teddy has gone off for a walk?
◆ Show teddy his name. Can you show him the 't' in his name?
◆ Who has a 't' in their name?
◆ Write a letter to teddy to invite him to come in and see us.
◆ Role-play area: 'Goldilocks and the three bears.'
◆ Stories:
  ◆ *Bear*
  ◆ *The Idle Bear*
  ◆ *I'm Coming to Get You*
  ◆ *My Friend Bear*
  ◆ *Small Bear Lost*
  ◆ *We're Going on a Bear Hunt*

Creative development

◆ *Activity plan: Make a room for teddy to play in (p. 227)*
◆ Role-play: Teddy bears' picnic.
◆ Observational drawing of teddy bears.
◆ Let's make up some songs for teddy.
◆ Teddy is hiding – can you help find him?
◆ Dress teddy up.
◆ Going on a bear hunt.

Physical development

◆ *Activity plan: Round and round the garden – teddy game (p. 226)*
◆ Take teddy for a ride or a walk.
◆ We're going on a bear hunt (follow the instructions in the story).
◆ Teddy likes bouncing on the parachute.
◆ Follow my leader (teddy).
◆ Take teddy round the obstacle course.

Knowledge and understanding of the world

◆ *Activity plan: Teddy's day with us (p. 225)*
◆ Can you take this little teddy on a ride in the programmable toy?
◆ Which of these is the oldest teddy?
◆ Display: Teddy at home with me.
◆ Take teddy home with you – take a photo of where he has been.
◆ Make some porridge for the three bears.

Mathematical development

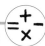

◆ *Activity plan: Put a teddy bear next to a friend (p. 224)*
◆ Order the teddy bears according to size.
◆ How many teddy bears can fit in this area?
◆ Let's count and label teddy's favourite toys.
◆ Sort teddy bears according to height, colour, ribbons.
◆ How many teddies in this feely bag – one, two, three or more?
◆ 'Goldilocks and the Three Bears' – can you lay out the table for the bears?
◆ Story: *Bear in a Square*

Activity plans for the theme 'teddy bears'

I *This is the Bear and the Scary Night* by Sarah Hayes

This is the story of a bear who was left behind in a park and was scared of the dark, but it has a lovely ending.

Specific resources

◆ teddy   ◆ story book   ◆ blue jumper (like the one in the story)

Key learning intentions

This activity helps children talk about moments when they have felt afraid or lost. It should also help them to think about what they should do if they become separated from the adults they are with while they are out.

Links to Foundation Stage curriculum

Area of learning	Aspects of learning	Curriculum guidance page
Personal, social and emotional development	Disposition and attitudes Self-confidence and self-esteem Making relationships Behaviour and self-control	32 34 36 38
Communication, language and literacy	Language for communication Language for thinking Reading	48, 50, 52, 54 56–8 62
Creative development	Imagination	124

Ideas for organising the activity

This book needs to be read with pairs or very small groups at first so that children can talk about the storyline. Focus them on talking about feeling lost or frightened.

Use this as an opportunity to talk to children about what they should do if ever they became separated from adults when they were out. After the story children can recreate and retell the story themselves with the props.

Extending and varying children's learning

◆ Ask the children to write a letter to teddy to tell him that he could always come to their house if he was lost.
◆ Paint pictures about times they have felt sad.
◆ Read the story again, concentrating on seeing if children can remember what happens next.

2 Guess what teddy can do 💬

This teddy is quite extraordinary – can you guess what he can do?

Specific resources
◆ teddy bear ◆ some props if required

Key learning intentions

This activity is designed to help children learn to ask questions and to expand their vocabulary. Children should also be encouraged to 'draw and write' once they have completed the activity.

Links to Foundation Stage curriculum

Area of learning	Aspects of learning	Curriculum guidance page
Personal, social and emotional development	Disposition and attitudes Behaviour and self-control	32 38
Communication, language and literacy	Language for communication Language for thinking Writing	48, 50, 52, 54 56–8 64
Creative development	Imagination Responding to experiences, and expressing and communicating ideas	124 126

Ideas for organising the activity

Show teddy to a small group of children (no more than six, so that they can easily contribute and do not become restless). Tell the children that teddy turns out to be an extraordinary teddy. Can they guess what he can do? Begin by modelling the questions for them: 'Teddy, can you cook?' Teddy will either 'nod' yes or no! 'I wonder what else you can do!'

  If they seem to find this difficult, you may wish to put some props in a box. Each child takes out a prop, e.g. a swimsuit, and can then ask teddy if he swims. Once the activity has finished, ask them if they would like to write down what teddy can do, so that they do not forget. They may also wish to draw a picture of teddy and this can be amalgamated into a display entitled 'Our Super Ted – Look at what teddy can do!'

Extending and varying children's learning
◆ Encourage children to play with teddy and the props so that they can make up their own stories involving teddy.
◆ Count the number of things that teddy can do.
◆ Repeat the game but concentrate on foods that teddy eats.

3 Put a teddy bear next to a friend

Can you make sure that each teddy bear has a friend?

Specific resources
◆ about ten teddy bears or 'compare bears'

Key learning intentions

This activity helps develop the concept of pairs and may also help some children to talk about not having a friend. Children should learn positional language while doing this activity.

Links to Foundation Stage curriculum

Area of learning	Aspects of learning	Curriculum guidance page
Personal, social and emotional development	Disposition and attitudes Self-confidence and self-esteem Sense of community	32 34 42
Communication, language and literacy	Language for communication Language for thinking	48, 50, 52, 54 56–8
Mathematical development	Numbers as labels and for counting Calculating Shape, space and measures	74 76 78–80
Physical development	Using equipment Using tools and materials	112 114
Creative development	Imagination	124

Ideas for organising the activity

Put out a group of bears – you may decide to have an odd number. Ask individual children to put the bears in pairs. Are there enough bears for every bear to have a friend? What could you do if a bear has not got a friend?

   If they find this difficult, spread out three bears, leaving the others in a pile and say that each of these bears now needs a friend. Tell the child to take a bear from the pile to be a friend. Children usually enjoy this activity and often talk about friends. Develop the activity by asking them to put the bears 'side by side' or 'one in front of another' to develop their positional vocabulary. You should also encourage them to count the bears. Can they tell you a story about the bears meeting each other – what might they say to each other?

Extending and varying children's learning
◆ Encourage children to play with the bears.
◆ Ask the children if they could write a note from one bear to another.
◆ Ask children to place six or seven bears into a circle.
◆ Ask the children to group the bears into threes, fours or fives.
◆ Put out written numerals and ask children to put the right number of bears onto or next to the number.

4 Teddy's day with us

Today we have a special visitor. We shall be taking some photographs of his day with us to help us to remember. What do you think he will enjoy doing? We will have to look after him to make sure that he does not miss his mummy.

Specific resources

◆ teddy bear   ◆ camera

Key learning intentions

This activity encourages children to use language to recall and to help them think about their setting. It will also help them to talk about things that they enjoy doing in the setting and encourage their sense of caring for others

---

Links to Foundation Stage curriculum		
Area of learning	**Aspects of learning**	**Curriculum guidance page**
Personal, social and emotional development	Disposition and attitudes Self-confidence and self-esteem Making relationships Behaviour and self-control Sense of community	32 34 36 38 42
Communication, language and literacy	Language for communication Language for thinking	48, 50, 52, 54 56–8
Knowledge and understanding of the world	Sense of time Sense of place	94 96
Physical development	Sense of space Movement	104 106, 108

Ideas for organising the activity

Begin by showing the children the teddy bear and tell them that he has come to visit them. The length of his visit will depend on how many children there are in the setting, as children in pairs should show him around. Encourage them to explain what they are going to do with him, why he will like it and what he can or cannot do. With some children you may have teddy become 'sad' because he is missing his mother or 'angry' because he cannot have all the toys. Encourage them to explain to him what is happening.

Take photographs with children during his visit. When the photographs are developed, use them to help children sequence his visit. Teddy should write the children a thank-you letter after his visit and ask them if they would draw him some pictures or write him a note.

Extending and varying children's learning

◆ Ask the children to do some drawing or writing for teddy to take home.
◆ Encourage children to tell teddy any of the 'rules' of the setting.
◆ Ask the children to make teddy a bed so that he can have a nap if he gets tired.

◆ Ask the children if they can find any clothes that teddy may be able to put on.
◆ Send teddy home with children.
◆ Display the photographs of teddy's day on the board.

5 Round and round the garden – teddy game

Let's play a game where teddy goes for a walk, but he must only take the number of steps shown on the dice.

Specific resources
◆ large dice   ◆ mats or pieces of coloured card   ◆ chalked squares to use as steps

> **Key learning intentions**
> This activity helps children to count and use numbers whilst concentrating on their physical development.

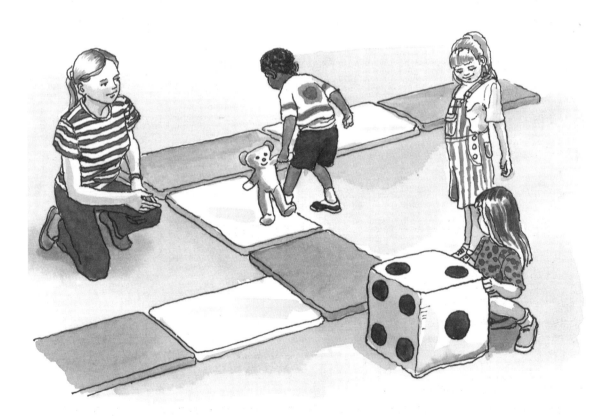

Teddy can only move the number of squares shown on the dice

Links to Foundation Stage curriculum		
Area of learning	**Aspects of learning**	**Curriculum guidance page**
Personal, social and emotional development	Disposition and attitudes Behaviour and self-control	32 38
Communication, language and literacy	Language for communication Language for thinking	48, 50, 52, 54 56–8
Mathematical development	Numbers as labels and for counting Calculating Shape, space and measures	74 76 78–80
Physical development	Sense of space Movement Using equipment	104 106, 108 112

Ideas for organising the activity

This game is ideal for small groups of children. Start by letting them run or walk around the space with their teddy bear before playing the game.

Each child has a teddy that they take for a 'walk' around the garden (squares of paper, mats or chalked squares). Teddy can only move the number of squares shown on the dice. This game can be made easier by using a dice with only the numbers 1, 2, and 3. If children are not ready to recognise numbers, the game can be adapted using colours, e.g. if a red is thrown on a dice, teddy moves to a red square.

Extending and varying children's learning

- Children develop their own 'garden' trail by changing the mats or paper around.
- Children sing the song 'Round and round the garden' and simply move with the teddy bear.
- Encourage children to make up a story about their teddy bear – where is he going?

6 Make a room for teddy to play in

Teddy wants us to make a room for him to play and sleep in. Here are some boxes and some things that you might like to use.

Specific resources

- boxes – large enough to fit teddy in
- card
- sticky tape
- fabrics
- paper
- staplers
- scissors
- bubble-wrap

Key learning intentions
Children will learn to use materials and tools whilst problem-solving and being creative.

Links to Foundation Stage curriculum		
Area of learning	**Aspects of learning**	**Curriculum guidance page**
Personal, social and emotional development	Disposition and attitudes	32
Communication, language and literacy	Language for communication Language for thinking	48, 50, 52, 54 56–8
Mathematical development	Shape, space and measures	78–80
Knowledge and understanding of the world	Designing and making skills Information and communication technology	90 92
Physical development	Using tools and materials	114
Creative development	Exploring media and materials Responding to experiences, and expressing and communicating ideas	120 126

Ideas for organising the activity

Explain to small groups or pairs of children that teddy wants a room where he can play and also rest. Encourage them to ask teddy questions about what he wants! (If possible, teddy might ask for a picture to be drawn on the computer to go in his room.)

Provide children with boxes, paper and free access to a choice of materials so that they can design a room for him. It is important that in this activity the adult supports rather than leads the children in any particular direction. Encourage them to measure the room they are creating against teddy.

Extending and varying children's learning

◆ Teddy may need other things in his room, e.g. a television or a bed!
◆ Teddy is very happy about his new room. Can you write for him to tell his mummy about his new room?
◆ Can you make a slide for teddy to go on?

Theme 19 Toys

This is a lovely theme as children can talk freely about their homes and what they enjoy doing as well as thinking about how toys work.

Inside the box on each area of learning below is a range of ideas for activities and stories on the theme of toys. You will find on the following pages a ready-made activity plan for the first idea listed in each box. In addition, all the stories mentioned are listed in the Booklist on pages 250–252.

Ideas to suggest to parents
◆ Show their child some of the toys that they had as children.
◆ Encourage their child to tidy away and sort out toys at home.
◆ Help their child to wash and look after toys at home, e.g. wash Lego, wipe seat of tricycles.
◆ Read books to their child about toys, e.g. *Old Bear, Spot's Toy Box*.

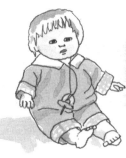

Personal, social and emotional development
◆ *Activity plan: Teddy's favourite toy* (p. 232)
◆ Looking after our toys – sorting, tidying and washing.
◆ Bring and buy sale or pack toys for other children.
◆ Share some of our toys – our own toy library.
◆ Show your favourite toy to a friend – why do you like it?
◆ Story: *Dogger*

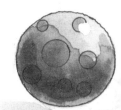

Communication, language and literacy
◆ *Activity plan: Role-play area: Toy shop* (p. 233)
◆ I am thinking of a toy – can you work out which one?
◆ Kim's game: Which toy have I taken?
◆ What toy is in the feely bag?
◆ Label boxes for toys.
◆ Interest table: Toys that begin with the letter 't', e.g. trains, tops.
◆ Stories:
  ◆ *Nothing*
  ◆ *Toby's Dolls House*
◆ Action rhyme: 'Here's a ball for baby' (*Round and Round the Garden*)

Creative development

◆ *Activity plan: Make some items for the doll's house (p. 238)*

◆ Move to the music – robots, teddies, wind-up toys – they all come out of the toy box.

◆ Make a 'Jack-in-the-box' toy.

◆ Draw/paint a favourite toy.

◆ Small world play – doll's house.

◆ Make your own toy box.

Physical development

◆ *Activity plan: Parachute games (p. 237)*

◆ Play with wind-up toys.

◆ Push and pull toys.

◆ Treasure hunt – can you find the missing toys?

◆ Printing in the dough with cars.

Knowledge and understanding of the world

◆ *Activity plan: Can you make this toy work? (p. 236)*

◆ Sort toys – which ones make music?

◆ Sort toys into groups.

◆ What are these toys made of – are they soft, hard?

◆ Remote-controlled toys – what can you make them do?

◆ Design and make a game.

◆ Old toys and new toys.

◆ Display: Our favourite toys.

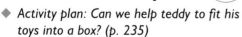

Mathematical development

◆ *Activity plan: Can we help teddy to fit his toys into a box? (p. 235)*

◆ Toys that are larger than my hand.

◆ Which toys are the heaviest?

◆ Which car will roll the furthest?

◆ How many toys will fit in this box?

◆ What does this toy balance with?

◆ Count toys – how many on this tray?

Activity plans for the theme 'toys'

I Teddy's favourite toy

Look what teddy has brought in. I think that this is his favourite and special toy.

Specific resources

◆ teddy and a small toy
◆ paper and pencils
◆ materials such as boxes, so that children can make a special box or place for the toy

---

Key learning intentions
This activity helps children understand why some toys are special and cannot be shared with others.

Links to Foundation Stage curriculum

Area of learning	Aspects of learning	Curriculum guidance page
Personal, social and emotional development	Disposition and attitudes Behaviour and self-control Sense of community	32 38 42
Communication, language and literacy	Language for communication Language for thinking Reading Writing	48, 50, 52, 54 56–8 62 64
Mathematical development	Numbers as labels and for counting	74
Knowledge and understanding of the world	Exploration and investigation Sense of time Sense of place	86, 88 94 96
Physical development	Movement	106, 108
Creative development	Exploring media and materials Imagination Responding to experiences, and expressing and communicating ideas	120 124 126

Ideas for organising the activity

This activity works well with pairs of children or very small groups. Show teddy and his toy to the children. Use teddy to act as a stooge. Teddy tells the children that his toy is special. He has a letter from his mother to say that it is special. Show the children a simple worded letter, e.g. 'This is teddy's special toy.'

Encourage them to ask questions about his toy. How old is it? Who gave it to teddy? Tell them that teddy does not like other people taking his toy and playing with it, because it is his very special toy. Do they have toys like that? Talk about why some things are special and ask the children if they would like to find a way of making sure that teddy can keep his toy safe. Maybe they could make a box or find a safe place for his special toy. Encourage them to write a note for teddy to tell him where he should put his special toy. Perhaps they could make a label for it.

Extending and varying children's learning

◆ Children work out a special place in the setting for putting special toys.
◆ Children write their names so that they can put labels on their special toys.
◆ Use teddy's special toy to help children think about toys that are larger or smaller.
◆ Read *Dogger* about a special toy that was sold by mistake.

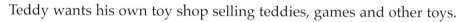

2 Role-play area: Toy shop

Teddy wants his own toy shop selling teddies, games and other toys.

Specific resources

◆ toys
◆ books
◆ play cheques
◆ boxes
◆ labels
◆ notepads

◆ games
◆ cash till
◆ calculator
◆ wrapping paper
◆ pencils
◆ cards with numerals

◆ cuddly toys
◆ play money
◆ bags
◆ scissors
◆ paper

> **Key learning intentions**
> This activity is designed to develop children's language, social skills and awareness of number.

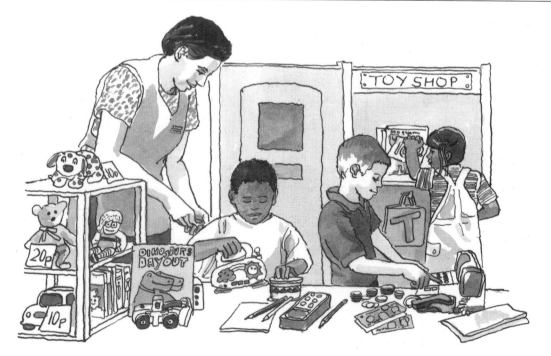

Encourage them to use the calculator and cash till to enjoy playing with numbers

Links to Foundation Stage curriculum		
Area of learning	**Aspects of learning**	**Curriculum guidance page**
Personal, social and emotional development	Disposition and attitudes Self-confidence and self-esteem Making relationships Behaviour and self-control Self-care Sense of community	32 34 36 38 40 42
Communication, language and literacy	Language for communication Language for thinking Reading Writing Handwriting	48, 50, 52, 54 56–8 62 64 66
Mathematical development	Numbers as labels and for counting Calculating Shape, space and measures	74 76 78–80
Knowledge and understanding of the world	Exploration and investigation Designing and making skills Information and communication technology Sense of place	86, 88 90 92 96
Physical development	Sense of space Movement Using tools and materials	104 106, 108 114
Creative development	Exploring media and materials Imagination Responding to experiences, and expressing and communicating ideas	120 124 126

Ideas for organising the activity

Ask children if they would like to help make a toy shop. Ask them to think of a list of things that would need to go in a toy shop.

Working with small groups, begin to prepare the toy shop. Encourage the children to select the resources that they think will be important. Ask them to produce labels and stick numbers on toys so that the prices will be available.

Once the role-play area has been set up, role model the language that will be useful by playing with the children. Encourage them to use the calculator and cash till to enjoy using numbers. This activity is a good opportunity for children to think about the 'rules' for their own toy shop, e.g. it must be kept tidy!

Extending and varying children's learning

◆ Visit a real toy shop.
◆ Ask children to 'draw' a plan of the toy shop.
◆ Put wrapping paper out so that children can wrap up toys.
◆ Provide boxes so that children can 'package' toys.
◆ Encourage children to make their own catalogue of favourite toys.

3 Can we help teddy to fit his toys into a box?

Here are some small toys. Which box would be the best box for teddy to put them in?

Specific resources

- teddy
- crayons
- small toys, e.g. small world people, toy cars
- three boxes of different sizes
- pencils
- paper

> ### Key learning intentions
> This activity helps children to use shapes, to measure and also to count. It will also provide an opportunity for children to 'write'.

Links to Foundation Stage curriculum		
Area of learning	**Aspects of learning**	**Curriculum guidance page**
Personal, social and emotional development	Disposition and attitudes Self-care	32 40
Communication, language and literacy	Language for communication Language for thinking Linking sounds with letters Reading Writing Handwriting	48, 50, 52, 54 56–8 60 62 64 66
Mathematical development	Numbers as labels and for counting Calculating Shape, space and measures	74 76 78–80
Knowledge and understanding of the world	Exploration and investigation	86, 88
Physical development	Movement Using tools and materials	106, 108 114
Creative development	Exploring media and materials	120

Ideas for organising the activity

This activity works well with individual children or pairs. Begin with a note from teddy asking if the children could help him to find a suitable box for his toys. Show them teddy, his boxes and his toys. Encourage them to talk about the toys. Are there any toys that are similar to ones they have? How many toys does teddy have?

Ask the children to work out which is the best box. Tell them to explain to teddy why they think one box is better than another. Ask them if they could write a note to teddy to remind him which box he should use.

Extending and varying children's learning

- Decorate the box for teddy.
- Make a list of teddy's toys so that he does not forget what he has.
- Clean teddy's toys.

4 Can you make this toy work?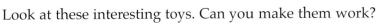

Look at these interesting toys. Can you make them work?

Specific resources

◆ a range of mechanical or remote-controlled toys – wind up, push down, pop up, etc.

Key learning intentions
This activity is designed to develop children's curiosity and interest in how things work.

Links to Foundation Stage curriculum

Area of learning	Aspects of learning	Curriculum guidance page
Personal, social and emotional development	Disposition and attitudes Behaviour and self-control Self-care	32 38 40
Communication, language and literacy	Language for communication Language for thinking Reading Writing Handwriting	48, 50, 52, 54 56–8 62 64 66
Mathematical development	Numbers as labels and for counting Calculating Shape, space and measures	74 76 78–80
Knowledge and understanding of the world	Exploration and investigation Designing and making skills Information and communication technology	86, 88 90 92
Physical development	Movement Using equipment Using tools and materials	106, 108 112 114
Creative development	Exploring media and materials	120

Ideas for organising the activity

This activity works well with individuals or pairs of children so that they can talk freely. Begin by putting out a range of toys – wind up, push down, pop up, etc. Ask the children if they can tell you how they work. If possible, choose some toys that can be taken apart with a screwdriver so that children can look inside – although this would need to be carefully supervised. Encourage the children to consider what the toys are made of.

Extending and varying children's learning

◆ Use a teddy as a stooge – can the children explain to him how the toys work?
◆ Can the children find other similar toys?
◆ Which toys are the children's favourites?

5 Parachute games

Come and play some toy games with the parachute.

Specific resources

◆ parachute   ◆ balls   ◆ cuddly toy
◆ tape recorder that children can operate   ◆ taped music with a strong beat

---

Key learning intentions
This activity is designed to help children's gross and locomotive skills.

Links to Foundation Stage curriculum

Area of learning	Aspects of learning	Curriculum guidance page
Personal, social and emotional development	Disposition and attitudes Behaviour and self-control Sense of community	32 36 42
Communication, language and literacy	Language for communication Language for thinking	48, 50, 52, 54 56–8
Mathematical development	Numbers as labels and for counting Shape, space and measures	74 78–80
Knowledge and understanding of the world	Information and communication technology	92
Physical development	Sense of space Movement Using equipment Using tools and materials	104 106, 108 112 114
Creative development	Music Imagination	122 124

Ideas for organising the activity

This activity works well with groups of eight or so children – enough for them each to have a 'handle' of a small parachute. Begin by putting on some music – can they move the parachute up and down in time to the music? Develop this by encouraging one child to stop the tape. When this happens the parachute has to quickly touch the floor!

Once this exploration of the parachute has taken place, choose one child to hide the cuddly toy under the parachute. The others take it in turns to find it. The parachute can be gently lifted up and down at this point. Finally, as a game, every child is told that they are either jigsaws, games or balls. When their name is called out they have to run around the circle and then come back to their place.

Extending and varying children's learning

◆ Play a game where a ball is put onto the parachute – can they keep it on top of the parachute?
◆ Play a game where several toys are hidden under the parachute and children have to find them by feeling for them on top of the parachute.

6 Make some items for the doll's house

Look at the doll's house. Can we make some things for it?

Specific resources

◆ small boxes   ◆ matchboxes   ◆ glue   ◆ scissors   ◆ stapler
◆ materials such as fabric, straws, pipe cleaners, lace, butterfly clips, wood, wallpaper

---

Key learning intentions
This activity is designed to develop children's ability to design and make items of their choice.

Links to Foundation Stage curriculum

Area of learning	Aspects of learning	Curriculum guidance page
Personal, social and emotional development	Disposition and attitudes Self-confidence and self-esteem Making relationships Behaviour and self-control Self-care Sense of community	32 34 36 38 40 42
Communication, language and literacy	Language for communication Language for thinking Reading Writing Handwriting	48, 50, 52, 54 56–8 62 64 66
Mathematical development	Numbers as labels and for counting Shape, space and measures	74 78–80
Knowledge and understanding of the world	Exploration and investigation Designing and making skills	86, 88 90
Physical development	Movement Using equipment Using tools and materials	106, 108 112 114
Creative development	Exploring media and materials Imagination Responding to experiences, and expressing and communicating ideas	120 124 126

Ideas for organising the activity

This activity requires close adult supervision, so consider working with individuals or pairs. Put out the doll's house, or if a doll's house is not available, put out some shoeboxes that could become rooms.

Ask the children what they think the doll's house needs, e.g. carpet, pictures, cupboards, tables. Show them the range of materials available and encourage them to think about how they could be used. It is important to remember that the role of the adult in this type of activity is to support rather than direct children. This allows children to learn more effectively as well as giving them a stronger sense of pride in their work. This activity should also be used as an opportunity to model positional vocabulary such as 'in front of', 'behind', 'next to'.

Health and safety
Make sure that staplers and other tools are used under supervision.

Extending and varying children's learning
◆ Each child could make their own room from a shoebox or similar.
◆ The children could make a mini garden for the dolls.
◆ Children could make larger items for their own home corner.

Theme 20 Water

This is an excellent starting point as many everyday activities involve water. Children can also start to notice the features of water, e.g. ice, steam, water on windows, etc. Water may also lead to themes such as weather, washing and boats.

Inside the box on each area of learning below is a range of ideas for activities and stories on the theme of water. You will find on the following pages a ready-made activity plan for the first idea listed in each box. In addition, all the stories mentioned are listed in the Booklist on pages 250–252.

Ideas to suggest to parents
- Encourage their child to wash up with them.
- Point out the weather each day – see if their child can remember what it was like the day before.
- Encourage their child to wash their hands independently.

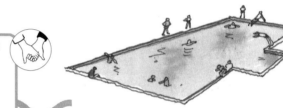

Personal, social and emotional development
- *Activity plan: What do we use water for? (p. 242)*
- Wash hands experiment.
- Making and pouring drinks.
- Making ice lollipops.

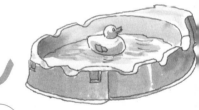

Communication, language and literacy
- *Activity plan: Mr Gumpy's Outing by John Burningham (p. 243)*
- Feely bag: Guess which item is in here – is it a sponge, toothbrush, rubber duck, soap?
- Stories:
  - *Meg at Sea*
  - *Mr McGee goes to Sea*
  - *There's a Hole in My Bucket*
  - *Umbrella Weather*
- Rhymes:
  - 'Five little ducks went swimming one day'
  - 'Five little speckled frogs'
  - 'Incey Wincey Spider'
- Pairs/picture lotto – pictures of weather.
- Kim's game: A tray of items associated with water – which one has been taken away?
- Your own weather diary.

Creative development

- ◆ *Activity plan: Making water shakers (p. 248)*
- ◆ Marbling – water and inks.
- ◆ Collage – mixing blues and greens.
- ◆ Bubbling painting.
- ◆ Painting on damp paper.
- ◆ Can you use the shakers to make rain sounds?
- ◆ Role play: Umbrellas, wellington boots, raincoats.

Physical development

- ◆ *Activity plan: Making and blowing bubbles (p. 246)*
- ◆ How much water can you wring out?
- ◆ Sponges in the water tray – can you squeeze them out?
- ◆ Can you pour this water into a small bottle?
- ◆ Painting walls with rollers, brushes and water.
- ◆ Catching bubbles.

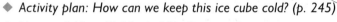

Knowledge and understanding of the world

- ◆ *Activity plan: How can we keep this ice cube cold? (p. 245)*
- ◆ How quickly will this puddle disappear?
- ◆ Which fabric will absorb the most water?
- ◆ Soil, sand or salt – which one will dissolve?
- ◆ Make a rain gauge.
- ◆ Sorting objects that float, submerge and sink.
- ◆ Making boats.
- ◆ Where can we find water in this area?
- ◆ Let's look at what happens when we put this bottle of water into the freezer.
- ◆ Funnels and tubing in the water tray – how does the funnel work?

Mathematical development
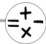

- ◆ *Activity plan: Floating frogs game (p. 244)*
- ◆ Which of these bottles of water weighs the most?
- ◆ Ordering bottles of water according to quantity.
- ◆ How many ice cubes will fit in this cup?
- ◆ How many scoops of water are need to fill …?
- ◆ Sinking the boat – throw a dice, put the number of teaspoons of water into the boat – who will be the one to sink it?

Activity plans for the theme of 'water'

1 What do we use water for?

What have you used water for today? Why is it important?

Specific resources

◆ paper   ◆ magazine   ◆ photos   ◆ materials for drawing and painting

---

Key learning intentions

This activity encourages children to think about the many uses of water that they see in their lives. It may be an opportunity to bring in the use of water for religious purposes such as baptism, washing before prayer, etc. if this is a part of children's lives.

Links to Foundation Stage curriculum

Area of learning	Aspects of learning	Curriculum guidance page
Personal, social and emotional development	Disposition and attitudes Self-confidence and self-esteem Sense of community	32 34 42
Communication, language and literacy	Language for communication Language for thinking Reading Writing Handwriting	48, 50, 52, 54 56–8 62 64 66
Knowledge and understanding of the world	Sense of time Sense of place Cultures and beliefs	94 96 98
Physical development	Using equipment Using tools and materials	112 114
Creative development	Exploring media and materials Responding to experiences, and expressing and communicating ideas	120 126

Ideas for organising the activity

With individuals or small groups of children, ask them when they use water in their homes and also when water is used in the setting. Ask them if they would like to find a picture or draw a picture of water being used. Encourage them to 'write' about what they have drawn. For most children, this will be 'mark making'. Paraphrase what the child has said or 'written' on a separate sheet of paper.

Pull together the children's work as a display. Parents can be asked if they have pictures or photographs of times when water was important in the family, e.g. holiday photos of a child in the swimming pool, or at a baptism.

Photographs can also be taken of children as they are washing their hands in the setting.

Extending and varying children's learning

◆ A further display could be produced – times when we wash our hands.
◆ An interest table could be used – things we use when we wash, e.g. towels, soap, rubber ducks!

2 *Mr Gumpy's Outing* by John Burningham

This is a story of a boating trip that went slightly wrong for Mr Gumpy and the animals.

Specific resources

◆ toy farm animals   ◆ a plastic or wooden boat

Key learning intentions
This activity is designed to encourage children's early reading and writing. The activity also provides an opportunity for children to recall and retell the story.

Links to Foundation Stage curriculum		
Area of learning	**Aspects of learning**	**Curriculum guidance page**
Personal, social and emotional development	Disposition and attitudes Behaviour and self-control	32 38
Communication, language and literacy	Language for communication Language for thinking Linking sounds and letters Writing Reading Handwriting	48, 50, 52, 54 56–8 60 62 64 66
Mathematical development	Numbers as labels and for counting	74
Physical development	Sense of space Movement	104 106, 108
Creative development	Imagination	124

Ideas for organising the activity

Begin by reading the story to a small group, e.g. four or six children. Use the props as you are reading it. Encourage the children to predict what is going to happen during the story. Follow up the story by leaving out the farm animals and the props so that children can 'play out' the story. Read the story to the children again but encourage the children to join in the refrains. Ask the children if they could 'write' a letter to the animals inviting them to come for a ride in the boat.

Extending and varying children's learning
◆ Put the props in the water tray.
◆ Ask the children to count the number of animals in the boat.
◆ Design a boat that will take many farm animals in the water tray.

3 Floating frogs game
Can you roll the dice and make your frog hop onto a different leaf?

Specific resources
◆ leaves or laminated pieces of card shaped like leaves
◆ plastic frogs or counters with frog faces on them
◆ receptacle for water, e.g. washing-up bowl, deep tray or water tray

---

Key learning intentions

This activity helps children to count and use numbers. It will need to be adapted carefully to the children's stage of number development. This game is also good to encourage positional language.

Links to Foundation Stage curriculum		
Area of learning	**Aspects of learning**	**Curriculum guidance page**
Personal, social and emotional development	Disposition and attitudes Behaviour and self-control	32 38
Communication, language and literacy	Language for communication Language for thinking	48, 50, 52, 54 56–8
Mathematical development	Numbers as labels and for counting Calculating Shape, space and measures	74 76 78–80
Knowledge and understanding of the world	Exploration and investigation	86, 88
Physical development	Movement Using equipment	106, 108 112

Ideas for organising the activity
This game is ideal for pairs or very small groups of children. The leaves are put onto the water and the child rolls the dice and then makes their frog hop from one leaf onto another. The game can end when the frog has leapt onto every leaf, although many variations of this game are possible. Dice can be altered so that it is only possible to roll either a 1 or a 2. Very young children may simply want to play with the water, leaves and frogs, and should be encouraged to do so!